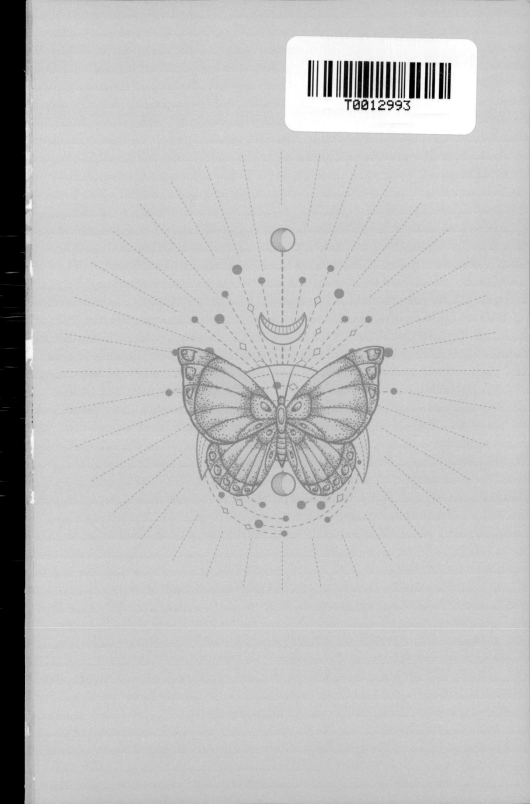

Praise for

YOU ARE MORE THAN YOU THINK YOU ARE

"I have learned so much from Kimberly's teachings for more than a decade, and this book is a life-changing read for creating more peace in your life."

— **Drew Barrymore**

"This book is an engaging, inspiring, and helpful guide to resurrecting your soul so you can embrace who you are truly meant to be. The time to tune into the glory and power of the True Self is now."

— **Deepak Chopra**, *New York Times* **best-selling author**

"You Are More Than You Think You Are is an intriguing and valuable practical guide that uniquely meshes ancient Eastern wisdom with the supportive science of mental wellness. No matter where you are in your personal journey, this book helps enhance your emotional resilience and let go of blocks that keep you from sustaining a positive, healthy perspective on life."

— **Dan Buettner**, **#1** *New York Times* **best-selling author, National Geographic Fellow, and founder of the Blue Zones**

"Kimberly Snyder is one of the most vibrant spiritual writers of the day. This book will not only inspire you to see beyond your limitations, it will draw you ever closer to your True Self, that inner place of transcendent beauty, personal power, and infinite potential."

— **Gary Jansen**, **award-winning author of** *MicroShifts*

"You Are More Than You Think You Are *is an empowering guide into awakening the conscious and fearless warrior that lies within us all. Kimberly thoughtfully weaves together ancient teachings, science, inspiring personal stories, and daily practices that give the reader a roadmap to harnessing the power of living from the True Self."*

— Dr. Shefali Tsabary, *New York Times* best-selling author and clinical psychologist

"In You Are More Than You Think You Are, *Kimberly Snyder takes you on a journey to break through all the stories, shame, and blockages that have stopped you from being the light that you are. Step-by-step you are guided to see that love is not something you go searching for, but more so something that is already here within you. I was moved by the vulnerability and strength held within this book."*

— Kyle Gray, best-selling author of *Raise Your Vibration* and *Angel Prayers*

"The wisdom of India has guided millions in the quest to discover who and what they really are. No one did more to foster that East-West transmission than Paramahansa Yogananda, and this wise, user-friendly book shows exactly how to use his powerful teachings to make our lives deeper, happier, and more fulfilling."

— Philip Goldberg, author of *The Life of Yogananda* and *Spiritual Practice for Crazy Times*

"Truly empowering! Kimberly is addressing a very needed topic in her new book. I highly recommend this book if you want to learn how to embrace and love yourself."

— Dr. Karol Darsa, author of *The Trauma Map* and executive director of the Reconnect Center

"This book is an accessible guide in showing how ancient teachings can help create success, joy, and fulfillment in modern life."

— GT Dave, founder and CEO of GT's Living Foods

YOU ARE MORE THAN
YOU THINK YOU ARE

ALSO BY KIMBERLY SNYDER

The Beauty Detox Solution:
Eat Your Way to Radiant Skin,
Renewed Energy and the Body You've Always Wanted

The Beauty Detox Foods:
Discover the Top 50 Beauty Foods
that Will Transform Your Body
and Reveal a More Beautiful You

The Beauty Detox Power:
Nourish Your Mind and Body
for Weight Loss and Discover True Joy

Radical Beauty:
How to Transform Yourself from the Inside Out
(with Deepak Chopra, MD)

Recipes for Your Perfectly Imperfect Life:
Everyday Ways to Live and Eat for Health, Healing, and Happiness

YOU ARE MORE THAN YOU THINK YOU ARE

Practical Enlightenment for Everyday Life

KIMBERLY SNYDER

HAY HOUSE, INC.
Carlsbad, California • New York City
London • Sydney • New Delhi

Published in the United States by: Hay House, Inc.: www.hayhouse
.com® • *Published in Australia by:* Hay House Australia Pty. Ltd.: www
.hayhouse.com.au • *Published in the United Kingdom by:* Hay House
UK, Ltd.: www.hayhouse.co.uk • *Published in India by:* Hay House Publishers India: www.hayhouse.co.in

Project editor: Melody Guy • *Cover design:* Shubhani Sarkar
Interior design: Bryn Starr Best • *Illustrations*: Lindsay Carron

Cataloging-in-Publication Data is on file at the Library of Congress

Hardcover ISBN: 978-1-4019-6311-8

E-book ISBN: 978-1-4019-6312-5

Audiobook ISBN: 978-1-4019-6313-2

10 9 8 7 6 5 4 3 2
1st edition, January 2022

Printed in the United States of America

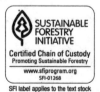

SUSTAINABLE
FORESTRY
INITIATIVE
Certified Chain of Custody
Promoting Sustainable Forestry
www.sfiprogram.org
SFI-01268

SFI label applies to the text stock

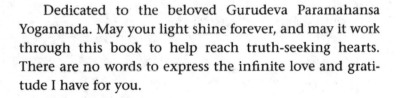

Dedicated to the beloved Gurudeva Paramahansa Yogananda. May your light shine forever, and may it work through this book to help reach truth-seeking hearts. There are no words to express the infinite love and gratitude I have for you.

And to you, dear reader. If you are reading this right now, you are one of the truth-seekers. May this book help to illuminate the truth of who you really are.

CONTENTS

PART I

Chapter 1: YOU ARE MORE THAN YOU THINK YOU ARE 3
Chapter 2: YOU ARE FEARLESSNESS 17
Chapter 3: YOU ARE A WARRIOR 33
Chapter 4: PRACTICE: Living in the Gaps 45
Chapter 5: YOU ARE LOVE 53
Chapter 6: YOU ARE WHOLE 69
Chapter 7: PRACTICE: Meditation, Part I: Foundation 87

PART II

Chapter 8:   YOU ARE PEACE 97
Chapter 9:   YOU ARE CONFIDENCE 109
Chapter 10: PRACTICE: Meditation, Part II: The Third Eye 123
Chapter 11: YOU ARE AN INTUITIVE BODY 129
Chapter 12: YOU ARE A POWERHOUSE 143
Chapter 13: PRACTICE: How to Supercharge Your Vitality 157
Chapter 14: YOU ARE BEAUTY 161

PART III

Chapter 15: YOU ARE MAGNETIC 171
Chapter 16: PRACTICE: How to Effectively Do Affirmations 183
Chapter 17: YOU ARE ABUNDANCE 191
Chapter 18: PRACTICE: Working with Mantra 207
Chapter 19: YOU ARE A CREATOR 213
Chapter 20: PRACTICE: Meditation,
             Part III: Expanding the Light 235
Chapter 21: YOU ARE THE TRUE SELF 243

Resources 247
Endnotes 249
Acknowledgments 259
About the Author 263

PART I

Chapter 1

YOU ARE MORE THAN
YOU THINK YOU ARE

*"You realize that all along, there was something
tremendous within you, and you did not know it."*

— PARAMAHANSA YOGANANDA[1]

DISCOVERING THE PATH

You are more than you think you are.

Those words can be challenging to hear. I know that firsthand, because I struggled with hearing them come out of my mother's mouth when I was growing up. I didn't believe them. In fact, I felt the opposite—that I was less, not more.

Like most young girls, and people in general really, I struggled with my self-esteem, doubted my intelligence, questioned my capabilities, and always wondered whether or not someone could love me. I carried a heaviness with me wherever I went. I felt anxious, I didn't sleep well, and I certainly didn't feel any sort of peace within myself. Nope, I was a bundle of nerves, spending a lot of my time focusing on my appearance, achievements, and what other people thought of me. All of this was pretty debilitating, to say the least.

But that all began to change one day when I entered a small bookstore in Rishikesh, India, when I was in my early 20s.

I had been backpacking for over two years at that point—part of a post-college journey to see and experience different cultures before jumping into the "real world" of work and responsibilities. Ultimately, that trip would span about three years and cover more than 50 countries. As you might imagine, I wanted to stay out of the "real world" as long as possible!

Back then, I was like a leaf blowing in the wind. I had no grand plan and mostly gravitated toward countries and places where I could eat, live, adventure, and experience life on a very small budget. India was a perfect place to do that. And Rishikesh, located at the foothills of the Himalayan Mountains (and called the Yoga Capital of the World), seemed like an interesting place to stretch a buck.

Dirty, dusty, and in need of a shower, I found an ashram where I could stay for a few dollars a day. There was a catch, however. To keep my rent low, I needed to commit to a two-week stay at the ashram, attend mandatory yoga and meditation classes, and do some service work in the communal areas.

It was the place where I got my first exposure to yoga. These classes were very traditional, focusing primarily on pranayama breathwork practices and meditation instead of the Americanized fitness-type yoga that was popular back at home (though at the time, I wouldn't have known any differently).

One day, looking to explore and get a break from all the quiet, I decided to leave the ashram community's insular world for the colorful and hectic world of Indian society outside the gates. I had no idea that day would forever change the course of my life.

Outside the garden wall, so to speak, monkeys and cows were wandering through the streets, and rickshaws decorated with shiny gold- and rainbow-colored photos of deities like Shiva and Rama were hurtling around every corner. The streets were lined with table stalls displaying rudraksha beads, little statues, fried street food, and orange flower garlands. As I was taking in all the exciting sights around me, I spotted a small spiritual bookstore with a slanted roof packed with hundreds of books on yoga and meditation. I wandered inside.

I browsed around for a moment or two. Then something strange happened. I felt like an invisible lasso pulled me over to a shelf that held some pale blue books with only the title and author's name printed in plain black writing on the cover. I opened one of the blue books (which thankfully were written in English) called *The Universality of Yoga*, by Paramahansa Yogananda. I had never heard of the writer, but I started to get goosebumps after reading just the first few words. And after reading for several minutes about the possibility of personal transformation, a "fire" sensation rushed up my spine. It wasn't heat per se, but more like a giant rush of energy that I had never felt before. "What is this?" I thought. I kept reading. The energy seemed to grow stronger. I couldn't put this little book down!

Yogananda's words felt like they were cutting through to my soul with his ideas of self-realization of who we really are, how to access a true inner power (whatever that was), the concept of "ever-new joy" and peace, and the interconnection of all things and all energy. I might have heard snippets of these subjects previously from hippie friends and wandering seekers on the road, but nothing like the truth bombs pouring through in just a few brief paragraphs as I leafed through the book. I immediately bought the small pamphlet for 30 rupees—and all the other books by Yogananda that were on the same shelf.

Those little books literally changed my life. I went from seeing things in a narrow, materialist way to having an expanded vision of a new reality. I felt like I had been putting on my T-shirt inside out for years, and suddenly I was shown how to flip it around. *Oh, the logo goes on the front!* Little did I know that that brief introduction to Yogananda's teachings would change everything in my life—not just for the better, but for the best.

Amazing. In just a few words, Yogananda had spoken to me, echoing the words of my mother:

You are more than you think you are.

And you, dear reader, are more than you think you are too. This book will help you to discover this for yourself.

ENLIGHTENMENT IS FREEDOM

Like many people, I have spent a considerable amount of time looking for something, never really knowing what that something was—acceptance, approval, a good boyfriend (eventually husband), money. But when I was fortunate enough to get each of these checklist items, I still felt like something was missing. In time and with the help of Yogananda, I realized that what I was seeking had to come from the inside, because nothing external, even the most wonderful things, could ever fill this void that all of us have.

It turns out I was seeking freedom all along. Freedom to be me, to feel light and joyful and peaceful, to live a life that feels good and authentic to me, to pursue what I would come to see as my life's work: namely, to serve others.

I discovered there was a spiritual word for the freedom I was seeking: *enlightenment*. It was enlightenment that helped me to see who I really was. And wow, it was more than I could ever have imagined.

Enlightenment seems like a big, daunting concept. Something achieved by only the very rare, privileged few like Buddha or Jesus. But actually, it's not so daunting.

To be *enlightened* means to be fully awake. Awake to the full flow of joy and love from within all the time! That's the place where Buddha and Jesus and Yogananda lived. And you and I can live from that place too.

Now, let's be honest: most of us probably aren't going to get to the top of that enlightenment mountain. I have no desire to hike to the summit of Mount Everest (29,035 feet), but I wouldn't mind making it to base camp (17,000 feet) to behold, up close, the glory of the Himalayas (that will be my next trip). But just getting on the *path* to enlightenment can give you, me, and all the rest of us ordinary folks a potentially massive upgrade to every aspect of our lives, including our health, relationships, careers, and even our finances.

And that's the point of this book—to offer you a path to enlightenment so that you, too, can experience that you are more than you ever thought you were. Enlightenment is about shining light on who you truly are. When the path is illuminated, you can see beyond your perceived limitations and tap into the power to discover that you are so much more than your current ideas about yourself.

Now, to unlock all that you can be—to have this experience of enlightenment that will change everything in your life for the better—you need to access the power of the True Self. Not the insecure, anxious self of social media images and fad diets who constantly compares yourself to others and then worries that you aren't good enough, but the real *you*, the unbounded *you* who has access to unlimited potential and possibilities.

THE TRUE SELF

So, what exactly is the True Self? Whole books could be written as an answer to this question. And in fact, much of Yogananda's vast writings explore this topic in depth. But for our purposes, allow me to offer this simple definition: *The True Self is the stable, loving, honest, courageous, peaceful, and creative intelligence that resides in each of us.* This intelligence is something we call Spirit, Love, Universal Consciousness, or God. It is the Divine part of who you are.

It's the you that you experience when all pistons are firing at the same time, when you are alert, focused, and happy to be alive. You know that feeling you get when, even if the whole freaking world is falling apart—you can't find your keys, the baby has crapped his pants, you just got a notice about your overdrawn checking account—you feel Zen and at peace? Well, that's an experience of the True Self.

Yogananda calls the True Self an acknowledgment of this Divine presence within you. He counsels, "Meditate every night . . . and sit in the temple of your soul, wherein the vast joy of God expands and engulfs this world, and you realize there is naught else but That. Then you will say: 'I am one with the eternal light of God.'"[2] That means that there is no separation between you and the powerful creative force that moves through all people and all creation.

And yet most of us don't feel very Divine at all. And there's a simple reason for that. We've forgotten how to be who we really are. We've fallen asleep at the wheel, so to speak, as we dangerously cruise with our eyes wide shut on a road of curves, potholes, and dangerous intersections. Discovering who you really are—realizing you are more than you think you are—entails waking up and taking control of your life by letting the True Self inside you take the wheel.

First, here's a short public service announcement: it's important to note before we go any further that Yogananda was a spiritual leader and writer. His books and talks always reference God. And yet he discussed God not as a way of promoting dogma or rules but as a pathway to "fulfilling your own highest potential." If, as you read further, the word *God* makes you feel uncomfortable, substitute it with the word *Love, Spirit, Universal Consciousness,* or *Higher Power.*

Ultimately, don't let names get in the way. The purpose of this book is to teach you to expand that True Self experience, so it's not something fleeting, but something you carry with you throughout the day.

Yogananda's teachings present a universal message that honors all religions, Eastern and Western. Whether you are a person of faith or an agnostic, yoga unites contrasting beliefs through love and connection. Yoga is not meant to replace or usurp your belief system. On the contrary, yoga is meant to enhance and elevate all parts of your life—mind, body, and definitely your soul.

Kriya Yoga

In the West, we are often taught to think that yoga is about learning how to do specific physical poses, or asanas. Maybe you've dipped your toe in—or have even become a die-hard regular at the yoga classes at your gym or neighborhood yoga studio. Either way, the physical part of yoga is just one small part of yoga (in types of yoga such as Hatha or Vinyasa Yoga), but that is not the kind of yoga we are talking about here.

Rather than just being about physical movement, yoga is a profound science amassing Eastern knowledge from thousands of years ago that can teach you to go beyond your self-imposed limitations, your fears, your lack of confidence. It contains the principles and secrets for helping you create your life, attracting what you want, reconstructing your body and your appearance, and achieving deep peace and joy in your day-to-day life experience.

Yogananda's teachings focus on Raja Yoga, the royal or highest path of yoga, which combines the essence of all the other branches of the comprehensive system of yoga. At the heart of Raja Yoga is the practice of definite scientific techniques of meditation and pranayama (life force control) known as Kriya Yoga. He called this form of yoga a "superhighway," the most effective road to experience the True Self within ourselves and the most effective path to Bliss. In 1920 Yogananda founded the Self-Realization Fellowship. Here he taught others how to build spiritual awareness through the Kriya Yoga science. And most importantly, he taught how you could use these practices in daily life.

Now, as I alluded to earlier, you might not feel expansive, loving, honest, courageous, peaceful, or creative right now. It's easy to get caught up in feeling anxious, separate, limited, and small. And chances are, if you are reading this book, you might think that something like developing a relationship with your True Self might not be significant or urgent at all. You might just be worrying about where your next paycheck may be coming from or whether or not a loved one has enough strength to brave a terrible illness. I get it. Focusing on everyday life is essential. I'm not saying it isn't. But, unequivocally, I can state that accessing the True Self is the most important thing you'll ever do. It will not only change your life—*it will save your life.*

How do I know? Because it saved my life. The reason I am so passionate about sharing Yogananda's teachings with you, which is the core of true yogic science, is because when I started to study and live these teachings, *everything* in my life drastically changed and vastly improved. It's when I started writing books and actually creating my dreams. Little by little, I went from being that anxious, insecure mess to feeling lighter and lighter and more and more joyful. Leaning on these teachings is how I got through many challenges and difficulties (which I will share with you in the upcoming pages), and how I started to feel truly happy in a sustainable, real way for the first time in my life. Not just the temporary highs of partying or fun events here and there, but simply in the everyday, ordinary moments.

I've always been passionate about sharing what has worked for me with my readers, which is why I've passed along my dietary philosophy and lifestyle principles in prior books. But this is the very first time I'm sharing with you my playbook for creating your most amazing, successful, truly joyful existence across *all* areas of your life.

I get asked all the time, "Well, how did you get started? And how did you create a business you love? How did you attract your soul mate? And how did you really get that healthy and have that much vitality?" I did it by accessing my soul power. **What you are going to read about in this book is going to teach you exactly how I was able to access my True Self and then apply what I learned to create all the best stuff in my life. Once I realized that I was more than I ever thought I was, I was able to create my dream life. You can too.**

When I look around, I see that Yogananda's teachings are needed more than ever. There's more anxiety, confusion, and discontent in the world than perhaps ever before. And with people's attention spans where they are, and with most of us getting our information and seeking answers in the fleeting, everyday news and social media, I felt like these real treasures, buried in dense books and texts that are not part of the news cycle, would pass most everyone by. And I just couldn't let that happen.

That is why I've gone through thousands of pages of Yogananda's writings and transcriptions to present some of his core teachings in a form that will be accessible and useful to you. I wanted to dig deep to present you with the real jewels of these teachings, which are not only useful but truly life changing. Ever since that day in Rishikesh, I have been living and breathing the teachings of Yogananda. He is my spiritual guru, and I credit these teachings with helping me create all the goodness in my life, including peace, joy, a beautiful family, and a deeply fulfilling career. And now I have the honor of sharing my teacher's wisdom with you.

You'll discover that you embody attributes that give you a lot of power to enact change and create a blissful, exciting, deeply fulfilling, and epic life. You just have to learn to *access* these qualities, which you will learn in each chapter of this book. It's not about "getting" any of these qualities, or enlightenment, but discovering that you already *are* them, and letting them come forward.

INTRODUCING PARAMAHANSA YOGANANDA

So who exactly is Yogananda? And why is he important?

Yogananda was a monk born in the late 1800s and was part of a lineage of exalted spiritual teachers bringing Kriya Yoga, which includes specific, ancient, and sacred techniques of meditation, back into the world. In 1920 he became one of India's first teachers to venture to the United States and spread yogic teachings to help people in the Western world. He returned to India only once after that, during which he met with and initiated Mahatma Gandhi into Kriya Yoga.

From when he was a young child, Yogananda was a spiritual prodigy. Both of his parents were disciples of the renowned yoga master Lahiri Mahasaya. When Yogananda was an infant, Yogananda's mother brought him to Lahiri Mahasaya, who gave him a blessing and foretold that one day he would be a great yoga guru. Yogananda received his monastic training from the revered Swami Sri Yukteswar Giri, who also told Yogananda that he had been chosen to bring the ancient science of Kriya Yoga to the West and worldwide.

His message was so powerful and resonated deeply with so many that people flocked everywhere he taught across the country. He is known as a *jagadguru*, a world teacher whose universal message serves as a source of blessing for the entire world and numerous cultures and religions alike. He spoke at many of the largest auditoriums in America at the time—from New York's Carnegie Hall to the Los Angeles Philharmonic Auditorium—packing them to their full capacity of thousands. He became so popular that he was invited to meet with the United States president at the time, Calvin Coolidge, and he influenced seekers from all walks of life over the decades, even after he left the body, including George Harrison of the Beatles, Elvis Presley, and Steve Jobs.

Hey, there is a reason that Yogananda's *Autobiography of a Yogi* was rumored to be the only book on Steve Jobs's iPad. Jobs knew that the principles Yogananda taught could help elevate his creative genius. And apparently, he felt so strongly about it that reports say he arranged to have a copy of *Autobiography of a Yogi* in a brown box given to the hundreds of people who attended his memorial service to serve as the last message Jobs wanted to leave to the world.

WHAT THIS BOOK WILL DO FOR *YOUR* LIFE

The purpose of this book is to allow me to share with you what I've learned and experienced through Yogananda's wisdom, and for you to take a ride with me on that superhighway to explore new ideas and arrive at a destination of new connection to who you really are. It is a destination of peace, health, happiness, and abundance. In short, I'm going to share with you the ancient Eastern teachings of how you, too, can live your most wonderful and meaningful life, the life of your dreams, by embracing the True Self.

Will this take work on your part? Absolutely, but no more work than you're probably doing right now in life. It just means a slight shift of focus. There's a lot out there about how to be more productive and to do more with less time. That's not what our focus here is. We're not talking about doing more. The core of Yogananda's teachings involve tapping into, using, and expanding your energy, or *prana*, the Sanskrit yogic term. Prana directs your health, purpose, relationships, and ability to manifest. Tap into prana, learn how to use it, and everything in your life will change for the better (we'll learn more about prana and how to direct it in Chapter 4).

You will learn how to tap into an inner power that will help you turn your dreams from fleeting hopes into reality. It will help make you more wise and more perceptive. You'll feel more awareness and depth. Colors will appear brighter, food will taste better, your intuition will explode, and you will find more of those states in your everyday life that we are all seeking: joy, inspiration, peace, and confidence. You will gain a lot more clarity across your whole life. Eventually, being in these states will become far more important and exciting than any specific achievement or material thing. But ironically, once you've tapped into your inner power, those achievements and material things will become easier to create too. It's a significant promise, but it's one I have experienced personally, so I know it's entirely possible for you.

A NOTE ON HOW TO USE THIS BOOK

Enlightenment is a state that must be experienced. We focus on this experience by contemplating and reflecting on the teachings in this book and practicing meditation.

True meditation, with the proper guidance and techniques, is the ultimate experience of truth, and the ultimate path to accessing the awesome power of your True Self.

There are specific meditations and various practices throughout this book for you to create that experiential knowing and go beyond intellectual understanding. I encourage you to get a journal for the self-reflections that go along with this book. Some of these reflections you will want to revisit periodically, like how you get physical check-ups from time to time, for as you continue to grow and evolve, more will keep coming into your awareness. When I reference our "practice," I am referring to meditation practice as well as learning to concentrate your energy within and the other practices called out here.

As we begin our journey together, please do read the book in the order that it is written, as the teachings are meant to build on the foundation of earlier ones. Part I lays the foundation for our book by addressing how to get past fear and other physical, emotional, and spiritual blockages, and opening up to love and purpose. **Part II** involves getting to know who you really are, and covers topics like peace, confidence, and true beauty. After Parts I and II, you are ready to create! This is what **Part III** is about: tapping into your true power to create your best stuff out in the world and manifest real and lasting abundance.

And remember that a beautiful, meaningful life is yours for the creating, right here, right now! As Yogananda taught, "For life's highest achievements, it is necessary to apply the untapped potentials of the human body and mind—powers that flow from the innermost essence of your being: your true Self or soul, made 'in the image of God.'"[3]

Chapter 2

YOU ARE FEARLESSNESS

"Darkness may reign in a cave for thousands of years, but bring in the light, and the darkness vanishes as though it had never been."

— PARAMAHANSA YOGANANDA[1]

As you read the words "you are fearlessness," you might think, "Not me! I have fear about not having enough money, ending up alone, getting some weird disease, and a million other things." I completely sympathize. But beneath all of these worries is the courageousness of your True Self that you can learn to tap into at any given moment.

Of course, some trepidation is healthy and is ingrained in who we are to keep us safe. We want to maintain a sensible fear of rabid-looking raccoons and driving too fast during a thunderstorm. But fear-based anxiety that stems from feelings of inadequacy—such as the fear of speaking your mind, fear of being misunderstood, or fear of failure—is all rooted in being disconnected from your True Self. When you feel you are not enough, when you feel that you are not lovable, it means you are identifying with your ego. This is the antithesis of your True Self.

Your ego is there for a reason; it unifies your experiences and gives them context. It's part of your humanness. But when the ego is out of whack (which most of our egos are), it takes on the role of a false self, a trickster, that likes to think it knows what it's talking about but is really reacting out of fear and not wisdom. The True Self is love and wholeness. Fear often comes from a feeling that we are missing something. The True Self misses nothing.

When you learn to embody fearlessness, life starts to take on a new dimension. You'll pursue what you want with your full power, instead of sabotaging yourself with doubts. Fearlessness lets you walk forward in a straight line through the forest of life, so to speak, instead of having to constantly stop and take side routes. When you embody this part of you, you will wake up to seeing life as an exciting adventure versus a frightening horror show.

FEARLESSNESS AS A SOUL QUALITY

In Yogananda's interpretation and commentary on one of the most important ancient scriptures from India, the Bhagavad Gita, he outlines a list of 26 soul qualities that allow human beings to reach their fullest potential. Guess which one is listed first? Fearlessness!

You might be surprised to find fearlessness as a primary spiritual quality to develop and call on in time of need. But Yogananda's wisdom teaches us that we can't possibly go deep into our connection with our True Self, with life, with our meditations, if we are riddled with fear and worry (in the upcoming chapters, we will go through specific steps for getting you started on your own meditation practice that are effective and easy to follow). Fear is a major obstacle to manifesting our dreams, but once our lives begin to flow, when we learn how to align with each now moment, we can let go of the past and obliterate any anxiety about the future.

To be limitless and experience union with Bliss, the goal of yoga, means you have to let go. Let go of the self-consciousness that so many of us experience. Let go of our reactions to the sensations and experiences that spring up around us at any given moment. Do we really have to harp on about the grumpy shopper who was rude to us in the grocery store all day long? Do we really have to react to every social media post that gets under our skin? I don't mean we should stick our fingers in our ears and wear a blindfold all day. You are going to keep sensing what is around you, but you don't have to take life so seriously.

You must also let go of putting all your faith and attention on what you can see with your physical eyes and what you do in your usual daily life. Fear can take hold only if you believe there isn't anything bigger than the everyday tumultuous storm of daily events that can toss you around. If all you believe in is this level of life, then sure, it can seem super scary. There are viruses, earthquakes, shifting economies, political unrest, global warming, and accidents. There's also the fear of not making it, of not having the right resources or skills to make your dreams happen, not to mention jealousy, which is fear of not having enough. There is fear of being alone. Fear of no one caring about you. Fear of having too much to do. Fear of success. Fear of failure.

All the "what if's" can feel like a lot, because they *are* a lot. We don't need to overstimulate our nervous system with all of this fear. It only leads to accelerated aging, disease, and death. There is supportive research, for instance, that finds that overstimulating the nervous system plays a role in the development of neuromuscular and neurological diseases.[2]

WHEN THE BAND-AIDS GET RIPPED OFF

One of the hardest things I have ever gone through was breaking up with my first son Emerson's father. My partner and I weren't moving forward in a way that was beneficial for either of us. Without going into detail, I knew that it was time to separate. It took an act of great faith to move out on my own with Emerson, who was not yet two years old, in tow. I had to trust that everything was going to be okay, because at the time it really did not feel like it. I used to cry in my closet after putting Emerson to bed, because my life was *so* not turning out the way I planned and wanted it to.

Breakups, especially if they involve a child, are beyond difficult (that is the understatement of the year). And I remember feeling shell-shocked at the time. I also started to panic that I may never find lasting love. One of my biggest fears (that I will discuss in the next section) started creeping back in—that I was not lovable. Especially as a single mom.

For about five months, following the advice of one of the monks I met with at the Self-Realization Fellowship (the organization Yogananda founded, which is centered around disseminating the Kriya Yoga teachings), I treated my home as a sacred place. I dove deep into rereading Yogananda's teachings, read spiritual scriptures like the Bhagavad Gita and the New Testament of the Bible, and

I meditated. Oh boy, did I meditate. It was my solace and my happy place.

In this rock bottom place of my life, I started to rise back up. And with that rising, came trust. Real trust, for the first time in my life. I began to trust the True Self within me. I trusted I could go through pretty much anything and be okay. It was then I began to realize that I could always look to that True Self for comfort and security, without having to seek it outside of myself. Even if my life at the time, as I saw it, was in shambles.

While my breakup with Emerson's dad was painful, I had to go through that crucible to meet my soul mate, Jon (I will share that story in just a bit too!), and experience the love I had always wanted but wasn't sure was possible for me. We moved to our dream house in the mountains and nature, which was much more aligned with my heart than the urban place where I had been living prior. But the biggest thing I learned from the whole experience was how to deeply connect to trust.

Whatever challenge you are facing, you can learn to trust that inner voice that is the True Self. You build that trust with getting to know and connect with the inner voice by spending time with it, which comes from your meditation practice and creating more stillness in your life. This trust will also allow the fearlessness in you to come forth, even if you've never thought of yourself in this way. In the moments that feel like the dark night of your soul, when things get really challenging, as they inevitably will in various ways for all of us, have faith that you will experience the bright morning of the soul too. It might take time, but if you can quiet the chatter in your mind, trust, and allow the True Self to do its job, you're going to need sunglasses when a new dawn awakens.

ACCESSING FEARLESSNESS

So where do we go to become more fearless? We go deeper. Meaning, we need to go inside, not outside. We need to move beyond thinking that the physical world is all that exists. There is something bigger, an invisible world that you can tap into and experience. If you don't believe me, then try this little experiment.

Imagine you just won the lottery. What would you do with all your winnings? How would you live? Where would you go? How would you live your life differently? Just imagine all the amazing things you could experience.

So, what just happened? If you're like most people, your body and mind reacted to this scenario. Maybe it brought a smile to your face, or your heart started racing because a lottery win could mean a radical, new, and awesome life. Maybe your mind exploded with endless opportunities to build the house of your dreams or create a nonprofit to help others.

But all of those scenarios were just your imagination having fun, and yet your body reacted.

In this tiny imagining you were able to tap into something you could not see. There *is* a deeper world you can access, a world where your inner gut feelings are the guides, not just your five senses, which are always tuned in to the outer world.

Fear can keep you thinking about what you are scared of, instead of focusing on what you want your life to be like and what you want to manifest. Fear keeps you from expanding and growing. It keeps you small because if you listen to it, you stick with what is predictable. Anything else might feel too big, scary, or . . . now here's a really annoying word . . . *unrealistic.*

And then there's the opposite: living a fearless life. Fearlessness means you go through life with faith. Faith in Spirit, faith in the True Self, faith in the greater force that is working through us and around us. To be fearless means that no matter what happens, you know that something very special and powerful has your back, so that you need to be neither overwhelmed nor paralyzed.

BRINGING THE FEAR INTO THE LIGHT

Now, I know I've spent the last few pages talking about getting rid of our fears, but it is important to explore the parts of yourself from which you may have disconnected, including your fears. This may seem a little contradictory. Perhaps, but as clichéd as it may sound, it is only by facing our fears that we have the chance to conquer them. You may not even be aware of some of your deep fears unless you go exploring within yourself, like rappelling into the cave of your subconscious.

For instance, when I started doing my practice, I had no idea yet as to what was at the root of so many of my life achievements and my motivations in general. Back in high school, I drove myself and those around me bananas because I wanted to be the captain of the track team, president of the school, and number one in my class. This heavily achievement-focused mindset pursued me into adulthood. I never looked at these goals as being fueled by fear until I started meditating.

It was through meditation—through the experience of focus and stillness—that I made a breakthrough. I mean, I cracked open and found that at the heart of my overachieving were deep fears: fear of rejection, fear of not being good enough, fear that I wasn't lovable, fear that I was never skinny enough, fear that my boobs were too small, fear that I would be left out because I wasn't cool enough, fear that I was not smart enough, fear that I wouldn't make my life a success, fear of not being taken seriously, fear of not even being seen because I was insignificant. I wanted people to pay attention to me, to praise me, because I didn't feel like I was someone whom others could find interesting, attractive, or intelligent. I feared I was nothing.

That's some dark shit. But part of the process of releasing fears is to probe through the muck that you have stored inside you.

Carl Jung, the Swiss psychiatrist and psychoanalyst, often discussed the idea that everyone has a shadow, which he said were all the unconscious, disowned parts of us. He believed we all tend to reject or remain ignorant of the parts of ourselves we don't like—and don't like to admit are part of us too.[3] We must muster the courage to look within ourselves, and really see. If we don't, then we aren't living from our True Selves, our true nature. Yogananda says, "True self-analysis is the greatest art of progress.[4]"

Take a deep breath, and let's go bravely looking into those shadows. We are shortly going to explore an important exercise that would benefit you to return to again and again, because the shadow is multidimensional. When we turn on a lamp in a room, the lamp not only illuminates what's in front of you, but the corners of the room as well. Maybe not as brightly, but we do see that there are things in the outer reaches that often need our attention too. The deeper we look into those shadows, the more we find them in there, until we get to the edge. Imagine that your shadow is a well. Psychiatrist Dr. David Hawkins says there is a bottom to the well. Eventually, if you keep doing the work, you will get to the bottom of the well of fear, darkness, and insecurity.

The parts of our practice—including meditation, pranayama, creating true stillness, concentrating our energy within—shed light on the shadow and bring it into focus. You may start to notice tendencies, reactions, triggers within yourself of which you were never consciously aware, and these will give you clues to keep digging down to the root of what fears are actually held in your shadow.

If you never take the time to examine your deepest fears, you won't truly begin to understand your motivations, your patterns of moving through the world, your very self. Maybe you keep attracting guys who cheat on you or treat you poorly, because deep down you have a fear that you aren't good enough for a quality man and that's all you deserve. Or maybe you don't go for the career you are so passionate about, because you have a fear you're not good enough to make it after all. Perhaps you might say that you *don't* want something (having kids, working as a full-time Pilates instructor, getting married, starting your own website, and so on), because you really *do* want that very thing, and you're fearful that you won't be able to get it. Maybe you keep getting cosmetic work done here and there because you can't shake this nagging fear that you're getting old and you're not going to find someone (or hold on to someone) who will love you.

If you can start to imagine what it would be like to be free from all of these fears, then you can start to imagine a new reality. When you even consider the possibility, it's the beginning of converting a potential into your reality.

Self-Reflection:
Getting the Fears Out of the Shadows

1. At the top of a fresh page in your journal, write, "My fears include:" and just start writing. Let your writing flow. Your list might include things like the fears of not having enough money to get through the year, getting old and saggy, the fear of never being able to have your own family, the fear of losing a loved one. Keep going.

2. Next, write at the top of the next page, "I am fearful of feeling:" and then again, create a list! This one might include fears around things like feeling left out (aka the notorious FOMO phenomenon), feeling lonely, feeling you never reached your full potential, feeling rejected, feeling stupid, and so on. As you go deeper (now or in a future repeated practice session), your list might also include not feeling loved or lovable, not feeling enough or good enough, not feeling important enough to be listened to or seen, and so on. Get them all out in the open!

3. Okay, you're doing great. Really! Nothing to fear here! Just one last list. On a third page, write, "Without any of these fears, I would feel:" Maybe you've never even considered what it would feel like to live without any fear. Seriously, what would you do, how would you act, how would you dance, sing, make love, work, hang out with your friends if you could not fail in any of your endeavors? How would you treat the people around you? How would you treat yourself? How would you wake up in the morning? How would you interact with those around you? Just let it all loose! Feel into it. Feel the liberation, the expansion, the confidence

that would come about without any of those fears. Close your eyes and really feel it.

4. Now, shred the first two pieces of paper up into tiny pieces, with the intention that you are now moving into the courageous, fearless place within your True Self. Keep the third in a safe place where you can access it, like in your journal or folded up on your altar (even if you don't call it that, this would be a place where you keep beloved objects, like framed photos).

5. Finally, commit to taking *one* step toward acting in a fearless way. Putting one thing in action, even if it is a small step, will start to make fearlessness a real energy in your life. It could be to research the field you want to move into for at least 20 minutes a day, or spend 30 minutes a day working on your brand-new business plan. Maybe it's signing up to take a salsa class (even though dancing in public feels like a nightmare to you!). Write that down in your journal, too, as a fresh commitment in the now: "I now commit to _____. Know that you have the power to create that new pattern of being fearless.

FEARLESSNESS IS NECESSARY TO FREEDOM

Fearlessness is the foundation of freedom, otherwise you will find yourself tiptoeing through life, staying in your little self-imposed cage. In freedom lies enlightenment: when you are freed from the ignorance that you have to be scared of life, scared to be yourself, scared that so many potential things are going to "get you," then and only then can your life expand into its most beautiful expression.

Let's face it—we live in a world with a lot of unknowns. There are countless things that could harm us. Be smart, be proactive, take charge, and at the same time, don't give a damn about these X factors. As the ideas in this book attest, you are capable of so much more than you believe. You are more than you think you are. You are a freaking miracle worker. Just don't be afraid to try to be one.

And one last note: You know why there aren't more miracles in the world today? Because how many of us wake up and say, I'm going to perform miracles in my life? I'm thinking mostly no one wakes up thinking that. Why? Because it's delusional? Perhaps. Or because we don't fully understand the crazy-ass power we have inside of us that can change our lives in an instant.

And this is the truth. Beyond your fears are your greatest dreams, your ability to live the best version of your life. Little by little, as you apply the wisdom and practices you will learn here, your fears will start to recede, and love and freedom will grow more and more abundantly in your life.

Practical Tips for Creating More Fearlessness in Your Life

1. **Surrender to the now.** *Surrender* is a word that gets tossed around a lot more these days as we Westerners have become more interested in seeking wisdom from the East. It's an interesting word because to some of us, surrender means we give up. But actually, surrender in the spiritual sense is more about merging. We merge with life; we merge our wants and desires with what is happening with

the now moment. We merge with Spirit's will instead of fighting or resisting.

The more we live in our moment-to-moment experience, instead of worrying about all the "what if's" in the future, the more we trust life, our True Self, and the more we can show up in a fearless way. Things are going to unfold, but it's our job to stay in inner harmony with what life brings. I know it can sound far easier to say than do, but don't worry, the more you commit to your meditations and practice, the easier your overall trust of life will get.

2. **Meditate.** I know this might seem repetitive, but the best things in life are repetitive, like breathing. So make your practice your new breathing. Meditation is the surest way to go below the surface of life and access your fearless True Self.

3. **Lean in.** When you feel the overwhelm of fear, close your eyes and locate where you feel it in your body. It might be in your gut, your heart, your throat, wherever. Focus on that area of your body and breathe in and out slowly. Don't think or analyze the fear, just fully feel it.

It may sound a bit cheesy, but the saying "What you resist persists" holds true. Let the fear be felt so that you can let it go, rather than trying to create resistance to it. After letting it run its course, which will probably take a few minutes (so long as you tune out your thoughts), you can open your eyes and *then* figure out the best action or step to take, which is sometimes to do nothing. If the feeling of fear comes back, do this again to release it from your body. This is what practice is all about: doing what helps us, over and over again.

4. **Fear vs. Truth and Wisdom Practice.** We all have access to the truth and wisdom inside of us, and this journaling exercise helps to bring it out of us. I was taught this exercise by Laura Pringle, a wonderful intuitive coach and healer.

First, write out your fear, and then let the Truth and Wisdom of the True Self from within you write back to that fear. Let the conversation keep playing out until your perspective of the fear feels quelled. At first, it might feel funny to have a conversation with yourself, but it can start to feel enormously empowering as you realize that you can be your own guide through your fear. Here's an example from my own journal:

Fear: *I'm worried people aren't going to like what I'm working on right now.*

Truth and Wisdom: *If you are authentic, then the right people will find you.*

Fear: *Yeah, but what if they don't?*

Truth and Wisdom: *Then they don't. At least you are authentic and living your truth, which is ultimately the most important. And let's be honest, we know they will find you, because all is energy and energy matches up.*

Fear: *True, but I'm scared of not being liked and accepted. I remember that feeling from when I was little.*

Truth and Wisdom: *You can like you. You can love you. And when you see yourself, others will too.*

Fear: Okay!

5. **Know you are never really alone.** This one may feel a bit mystical, but if it resonates with you, then use it. When you feel really fearful, close your eyes for a moment and create an intention of protection. You can simply imagine a presence of energy surrounding you, a white bubble of light around you, or a light inside of your heart that is walking with you. Maybe it's an image of a guide or an angel that is right there with you that feels personal to you. Choose the imagery that resonates best with you and go with that.

Chapter 3

YOU ARE A WARRIOR

"God sent you here for a purpose. . . . Realize how tremendously important that is! Do not allow the narrow ego to obstruct your attainment of an infinite goal."

— PARAMAHANSA YOGANANDA[1]

PEACE WARRIOR

We often think of warriors in mythological terms: strong men and women yielding bows or swords and seeking to right wrongs. But the idea of the warrior is something that is crucial and important to your life today.

You are a warrior.

You are someone who can draw on inner strength, overcome obstacles, and persevere. You can be a warrior for good, for love, for positive change, for the betterment of all, and for accomplishing worthwhile goals, especially goals that support your central purpose. Your expression of the warrior may be soft and gentle, yet still enormously powerful to stay focused and enact great change. The more you align your actions, natural talents, and best ideas around helping others (which we will discuss in Chapter 19), the more successful you will become.

Like a warrior, the True Self is courageous and unwavering, determined and fierce, focused and steady. In order to move through the trials and busyness of life, and to remain focused on moving further along the path to freedom, you need to access the True Self's warrior strength.

THE GREAT BATTLE OF LIFE

As noted earlier, the Bhagavad Gita is one of India's most important and inspirational ancient texts. It's about a great battle, which is really an extended metaphor for the great battle we are all waging every day: the battle of the mind. The Gita can be read as an exploration of the battles that go on in our heads, between the voices that support us and the voices that try to tear us down; the battle between our wisdom versus the pull of our senses and the ego.

In the story, the main character, Arjuna, represents you and me—us humans on the path to enlightenment and yet plagued with doubt, worry, and bad habits. It is these thoughts that often keep us from realizing the True Self within each of us. Arjuna, wanting to win in battle, receives counsel from Krishna, who represents the voice of the True Self.

One of the major themes of the Bhagavad Gita is about *dharma*, which roughly translates to our life purpose, our duty, or how we fit into the Divine plan of existence. Krishna counsels Arjuna to "fulfill his Kshatriya (warrior) duty to uphold dharma" through "selfless action." What does that mean? I'll go into more detail in a moment, but first I want to talk about a real-world warrior as an example.

I interviewed Ruth Zukerman for my podcast, and I was quite taken with her story, probably because I could relate to it so much. Ruth became a single mom when her twin daughters were six years old. She had to scramble to financially support herself and her girls. As she said, "There certainly was no money for babysitters!" Ruth had to figure stuff out. Up until this point in time, she had never held many full-time jobs. And she certainly had no business background. But she was a good dancer. She parlayed her knowledge of dance and general fitness along with her love of music to become a spin instructor. And not just a run-of-the-mill spin instructor, but one who would motivate and champion her students to new heights of awareness, strength, and endurance.

Fast forward five years. Ruth co-founds SoulCycle, an international spin-based boutique fitness studio with nearly 100 locations around the world at the height of its popularity. She was 48 at the time. Move ahead another four years and she becomes the co-founder of another fitness chain called Flywheel, a company she would sell for millions of dollars a few years later.

When I asked her about her success, she responded that she never focused on being inexperienced in business or considered that she might have missed the entrepreneur boat. She always felt incredibly connected to her students and wanted to inspire as many of them as possible. That was Ruth's purpose. To educate, motivate, and inspire people from all walks of life to embrace fitness and right thinking, and to help them achieve their dreams. Her goal in life was *to help others* meet their goals in life.

Everything else sprang from that chief purpose—from creating the right training manuals, to methodology, to fitness programming, and to the development of a company culture that made her brands miles above the rest. And the best part of this story? Ruth is incredibly warm and kind, and even though she focused on a business goal, she never lost focus of her daughters or stopped being there for them as a mom. She is the embodiment of a warm, heart-centered, kind, trustworthy warrior.

When Krishna advised Arjuna to uphold his dharma through selfless action, he was talking about doing what Ruth did. Keep your eye on what is important. Throw yourself into the din of battle and do not worry about results. When you do so, you allow the True Self to handle the daily battle of your life, while you can take care of the things and people you love.

YOUR PURPOSE

Each one of us is unique, and each one of us has a unique purpose. When you are aligned with your purpose, it means you are part of something bigger than yourself. Your purpose will then move you into action steps and move through you, and you end up having more energy to make your dreams happen. In fact, a lot of the "work" you do—whether it's baking, picking up the kids from school, running a business, plucking your eyebrows, or even spending time with the in-laws ceases to feel like work. It starts to feel like an extension of who you are, and what you are contributing to the world. When this happens, you know that you have opened the door to the True Self working through you.

This is why it's so important to have warrior vision. A warrior sees beyond what's in front of her eyes. A warrior is aware of everything around her. She sees in widescreen. Though it's important to tackle the task at hand, it's also important to pay attention to what's going on around you. In this day and age, in the 24-hour nonstop cycle of modern life, or warriorship, we need to realize that we aren't just going to battle for ourselves, but for those around us. When we work only for ourselves, it's far easier to quit and break down and get tired. Frustration takes hold and we feel depleted.

Bottom line: selfishness sucks. It doesn't make you truly happy; it doesn't energize you; and it makes your life small. You might have fun for a little while, but selfish people always end up alone and bitter. Think about it: Have you ever spent time around a truly selfish person? Hopefully, you didn't spend much time, because that shit gets old fast. Selfishness divides.

In order to grow your world, in order to really experience an epic life, you really do have to do what the warrior does, and that is to give your life away. It sounds counterintuitive. But consider this: the more love you give to others, the more you will get back. The more time you give to others, the more time you'll get back. The more you give, the more comes back to you. Now, you might not get that time back right away. You might not get love back from someone you give it to, but it does come back to you. Call it the universal law of reciprocity. Call it karma. Call it Bob. It doesn't matter. Give your life away and you get it back.

There's no scientific evidence for any of this, but there is plenty of anecdotal evidence all around us. Who are the happiest people? The ones who care only about themselves? I think not. It's those who live from a bigger place.

Why am I spending so much time on this? Because you may think your life's purpose is to create rocket ships or a new line of athletic wear or the best gluten-free cupcake on the West Coast, but **really your purpose is to serve others.** And that's what the great heroes do. That is what a warrior does. Rarely do warriors battle for themselves. A warrior fights for something bigger than the little self. The warrior stands for the True Self within herself and others, which is the highest and best version of all of us. It's your unique way of serving others in the world that makes up your unique purpose. It is only through the context of the collective, being part of the greater community around us, that we can feel that our lives are truly meaningful and directed by purpose.

In this way, we all have the same purpose and yet it's different at the same time. What do I mean by this? For all of us, our core purpose is to serve others, to help others in some way. It is by doing this that we ourselves expand and grow. We grow past our own limitations, and so we are also helping ourselves reach our highest potential and stretch to actualize our dreams. If we stay small and focused on ourselves, then we reinforce our limits. Yogananda was very clear about this: "To act with self-interest is to lose sight of the cosmic plan or will of God."[2]

Yet your purpose is unique to you because you have a unique energy that you bring into the world, and so it will get channeled into work and projects in a way that only you can do it. In other words, you can serve and help others in a unique way. In Chapter 19, YOU ARE A CREATOR, we're going to take a deep dive into your unique essence, but for now just let this idea start to sink in. You're here to serve in your own unique way.

Now, I'm not saying you must sacrifice your dreams. I'm not saying you have to give up the things you love. I've worked with too many people over the years who feel like they have given, given, given, and have never gotten anything back. They're angry, they're disappointed, and they often walk through life as if they have a dark cloud over them (sort of like Eeyore from Winnie the Pooh). I often think that the reason why this gloom seems to fall on certain people is because they could never get clear on their purpose and so they sacrificed who they were out of fear or confusion or loneliness. A warrior would never do that.

My purpose is also to serve others, as yours is too. My unique spin on it is to help others connect back to their True Selves and their True Beauty—the genuinely beautiful part of each of us that is far below the surface. I do this by helping as many people as I can feel good by teaching a holistic lifestyle that includes a focus on food, body, emotional well-being, and spiritual growth (what I call Solluna's Four Cornerstones of True Beauty and Wellness). I also raise my children as consciously as possible, strive to be a loving wife, friend, and member of the community. And that's ultimately why I've written this book: to help you discover and embrace your own purpose, and to remind you to let your inner warrior protect, guide, and defend your honor. I can't wait to hear more about *your* purpose in our community!

Self-Reflection: A Warrior's Purpose

Developing a warrior's purpose requires some real self-reflection. We have to dig past the layers of obligation; expectations of ourselves, family members, and other loved ones around us; limited beliefs; and fear. It requires you sitting with the questions that follow, writing them out in your journal, and then returning to them time and time again to hone and reflect. We go deeper into exploring this topic later in the book, but let's start here first:

1. What are you passionate about? What really lights you up?

2. Fill in the blank. When I look back at my life, I will be most proud of _____.

3. What are your unique gifts, or ways you do things, and how does that relate to your purpose of serving others?

4. If you had a billion dollars, what would you do with your time?

5. I love to help others _____.

DEVELOPING PERSEVERANCE

The great writer and poet Johann Wolfgang von Goethe aptly said, "In the realm of ideas everything depends on enthusiasm . . . in the real world all rests on perseverance." Warriors persevere. Maybe right now you're feeling a little tired of life. Maybe you feel like you've gotten your teeth kicked in a couple of times, so to speak. Maybe you've been laid off, a business plan has been derailed because of a pandemic, infidelity left you blind-sided, a health diagnosis left you reeling, your lovable middle schooler has morphed into a ranting teenager who hates your guts, or a romance has fizzled out for no other reason than the relationship had run its course. All of these things, and so many other ordinary and not-so-ordinary struggles, can be extremely challenging and disheartening.

Yet difficult doesn't mean bad. Nor does it mean failure. Just because something is tough doesn't mean it can't be beneficial to your life. In fact, it's the challenging moments in our lives that help to further define who we are. As Yoga-nanda says, "No matter how many times you fall down, get up with the determination to be victorious."[3]

One of the most important warrior perspectives you can develop is to focus your power on the present moment rather than on the past or the future. This can be tough to do, of course. We worry about past mistakes, perhaps, and how they might affect our life tomorrow. There's a part of us attuned to survival, and part of this survival instinct is to think about things that could harm us, which is why so many of us can become preoccupied with things we've already done and what could happen in the future. But you are meant to be more than a survivor. You are meant to flourish. You are meant to be far, far more.

LETTING THE PAST GO

Yet a critical element to success is to stop obsessing over your past failures. If you attach yourself to failures, you are aligning with happenings and occurrences. It's just another way of forgoing aligning with the True Self and instead aligning with an aspect of your small self, or your ego.

Essentially, to focus on your past is like stepping in dog poo, realizing you stepped in dog poo, walking back to make sure it was dog poo, and stepping in dog poo again. Repeat. All this does is wreck your shoes and make you smelly. You do the same thing when you relive your mistakes and disappointments over and over. Do you really want this energy in your life?

Let's be real: we have all failed at one time or another. In other words, we've all stepped in it. Yogananda describes the multiple times he went penniless when he was trying to support the Kriya Yoga work in the United States. "Every failure gives you the privilege of learning something new,"[4] he says. Yet he refused to give up, and ultimately, he found a way to succeed. And you can too. Make up your mind to succeed, learn and then let go of past mistakes, bring out the *warrior* in you, and you will become unstoppable.

Practical Tips for Being a Warrior in Your Life

1. **Organize your life.** Yogananda urges us to "methodize your life." A warrior is organized with his or her time, so he or she can maximize daily efforts and energy toward his or her purpose. I've always talked about the importance of creating a morning and evening practice, to consciously create a flow to how you start and end your day. If you are disorganized, you will waste a lot of time and energy. So, get organized, and also schedule time for your practice and meditations so they become as honored and important as your daily list of to-do's.

2. **Develop self-reliance.** Depend on your own
    inner strength. Never think you have to rely
    on someone else for your success. Sure, helpful
    contacts are important, but ultimately, it is your
    own valiant, consistent efforts—your smart
    actions—that take you where you want to go.

    Yogananda teaches us, "Be honorable
    enough never to hang on anyone else. You are a
    child of God. You have all the power necessary
    to take yourself where you want to go."[5]

3. **Develop patience.** This is not the easiest quality
    to develop, I have personally found, but along
    with willpower and intuition, this is important
    for success. Things don't always work out in the
    time frame that you want. It's important that
    you remain positive and focused, like a watchful
    warrior, knowing the difference between being
    patient and letting things slip by the wayside.
    Feel into the wisdom inside of you, in order to
    discern when to take action, when to gather
    information, and when to simply be.

4. **Work for something greater than yourself.** As
    I've mentioned, if you are working for yourself,
    it's far easier to quit and break down and get
    tired. But when you are part of something much
    larger, and your purpose includes dedicating
    your efforts to something much greater than
    yourself, you will find yourself blessed with
    infinitely more energy to get through the day.

5. **Write down your purpose and place it on your
    altar or other focal point.** I revisit my purpose

and the goals that align with it regularly, and I write them out on pieces of paper I fold up and place on my altar, either in a little bowl or underneath one of the statues, making sure it is peeking out so it catches my eye. By doing this, you keep your purpose as a focal point in your home and in your room.

Life gets busy and it's easy to let things slip, but don't let your purpose slip from your mind. Ideally, it's something you reflect on every day as a warrior. Look at your purpose like a Warrior's Code, a statement you live by every day. A statement that guides your decisions and keeps you rooted to your overall higher purpose as you move through life.

Chapter 4

PRACTICE:
Living in the Gaps

*"One cannot attain Self-realization
without breath mastery."*

— PARAMAHANSA YOGANANDA[1]

MORE ON PRANAYAMA

Working with the breath is not only the most basic and important of all life functions, but also one of the ways you can access the True Self to discover who you really are. In yoga, techniques for working with the breath are referred to as pranayama. The Sanskrit word *prana*, as noted earlier, translates to our life force, which controls all the body's systems and functions. So the practice of pranayama is all about directing your life force, this energy within you.

The more you can direct your life force, the more you can maintain and boost your health and overall energy, the more you can tap into more creative solutions and ideas, and the more you can feel centered and calm through all situations.

Research has found that focusing—concentrating—on your breath can boost gamma brain waves.[2] Why is this important? Gamma brain waves are associated with peak concentration and processing information,[3] as well as assisting to improve your memory and possibly preventing Alzheimer's.[4] Perhaps most exciting, elevating your gamma brain waves can improve your overall mood, keep you emotionally stable, and prevent you from feeling stressed out and depressed.[5] **Concentration and equanimity are key foundational qualities for creating greatness in your life.**

One of the best-known teachings in the *Yoga Sutras*, a 2,500-year-old guidebook written by the great Hindu sage Patanjali (it's notable that Kriya Yoga is twice mentioned in this ancient text), is *Yoga chitta vritti nirodha*. This translates loosely to "yoga is that which helps stop the mind stuff." Mind stuff, or vritti, translates to "whirlpool," the waves of thoughts and emotions that spin and spin and threaten to drown us mentally, psychologically, and spiritually. Pranayama, then, is the practice of calming the restlessness of the mind so you can access the peace that is at the center of your True Self. In other words, if your life isn't what you want it to be, I can almost guarantee that it's because you are not experiencing more peace in your life.

Don't worry, though, because you can learn to use your breath and meditations to calm yourself down. And by calming down all the spinning madness that whirls around in your brain, you will see significant changes in your life.

I'm not going to BS you. Meditation isn't easy at first, especially if you're someone like me, whose mind has a hard time sitting still. When I first started meditating, I used to squeeze my eyes shut so tightly that my nose would wrinkle up like a raisin. This was my futile attempt to try to keep from peeking at the time every 20 seconds. "Is this over yet?" That was my initial mantra! So it took time for me to bring my monkey mind under control. I can promise you that the more you meditate, the more you practice focusing on your breathing, the better things will get. Not just with the meditation, but with life!

In this beginning practice, you will learn to withdraw your attention from your five senses and all the messages they consistently bring to you. Though important for performing tasks in the world, like driving, cooking, or sensing the right temperature for your shower, the senses can be a distraction from connecting to the inner power within you. Are you going to fully turn off your senses? Of course not. We're just going to dial them back a little so that the True Self can have some time to speak.

ACCESSING AND EXPANDING THE GAPS

In the practices that follow, you will focus on following your breath. As you start to pay attention to your breath, you will find that it naturally starts to slow down. Imagine a child who's running all over a room. Now imagine a child's parent in the same room. At first the parent isn't paying attention to the kid, but then after a few minutes of juvenile chaos, the parent stops what she's doing and stares at her kid. What happens? It might take a minute or two, but something will eventually go off in the child's brain to slow down and to stop the disruptive behavior. Don't believe me? Cue up any episode of *Supernanny*, and you'll see Jo Frost use that technique like a charm. Well, following the breath is like that.

Focusing on the breath and the subsequent slowing down of the breath helps you disconnect from outer distractions, and this is a very good thing. Furthermore, it's great for your body and your health. Scientific research has found that slow breathing has significant positive effects on different systems in your body, including your cardiovascular, respiratory, and autonomic nervous systems.[6]

Now here's the most important part about focused breathing: just by watching the breath, not only will it start to slow, but the pause between the inhales and exhales will start becoming longer and longer. **It is in these gaps where the magic is! It is in these gaps where you can start to connect to the deepest parts of yourself. In the gap is peace. In the gap between thoughts is stillness. In the gaps is where you catch glimpses of your True Self waving to you as if to say, "Hi, remember me?"**

This might sound a little flighty and esoteric, but a simple question and answer might help to illustrate more fully what I'm talking about when I talk about the importance of gaps. Are you ready? Here's the question:

Q: What happens when you don't have gaps in your life?

A:Thisiswhathappenswhenyoudon'thavegapsinyourlifethingsgetconfusingandtheydon'tmakesense lifeisinefficentandmessyandit'sreallydifficulttoreadanswerslikethisone.

See my point? Gaps give us order. If we didn't have gaps between words, all of those letters wouldn't make a lot of sense. Gaps help to organize us. Gaps allow us to take breaths. Gaps exist between thoughts and words. Gaps exist in music; if we didn't have gaps, all music would sound like cacophonous madness. There is the gap between morning and night. The gap we call sleep is that stage between all of our waking hours. We need gaps—we need those periods of rest—and we need to learn to focus on the power that lies within them.

In the gaps that exist between breaths is the space where Yogananda says you can access "soul awareness." It's a state where you can calm your heart, redirect energy from your senses, hone your concentration, and connect with the Spirit within you that is your True Self. To create this state, Yogananda says that drawing the energy inward and slowing your breath are necessary.

The medulla oblongata is the part of your brain at the base of your skull where the yogis believe you can pull in and access more energy. This energy is believed to sustain everything and is intelligent in nature, meaning that it is self-organizing, coordinated, and can take on infinite forms depending on how it needs to be used. It is the energy that is fuel for your life and for your body. The fuel that can slow down aging and empower your goals and dreams.

Scientists agree the medulla is critically important to many of the basic autonomic bodily functions that we usually take for granted, including our heartbeat, breathing, sneezing, swallowing, and so on. It's been discovered that the neurons in the medulla are largely responsible for the overall stability of our internal environment, which includes the gases, nutrients, ions, and plasma that are necessary for maintaining life.[7]

Bottom line: pay attention to the gaps!

Expanding the Gaps Practice

1. Take a comfortable seat and lift your spine upright so that it's fairly straight from your seat to the crown of your head. Make sure your head isn't jutting forward—a common occurrence in the modern smartphone-saturated world!

2. Next, place all your concentration on your breath. Simply watch your breath flow in naturally with your inhales, and flow out naturally with your exhales. Don't try to control it, count it, or manipulate it to be any kind of pattern. Just watch it.

3. It may be helpful for your mind to concentrate on a simple mantra, like "let go," to stop the mind from wandering and focus on the breathing. So when you inhale, you breathe in "let," and when you exhale, you breathe out "go." Don't try to time the breath to the mantra, however; let the mantra follow the breath.

4. Start to pay extra attention, as you get going, to the gaps, the spaces *between* your inhales and exhales, where your breath takes a natural pause. As you pay attention to your breath, it will start to naturally slow down, and the gaps between inhales and exhales will start to expand. Again, don't try to force this. Just observe. Simply watch it and be calm.

5. Try to keep your body very still, and don't pay any attention to the little micromovements of your body. Just breathe as softly and with as little physical movement as possible. Never

hold your breath with force or refuse to take a
breath if you need one. This should feel like a
natural flow.

6. If your mind wanders, calmly but consistently
    come back to simply observing the breath.
    (Over time it definitely becomes easier to keep
    the mind from wandering! I used to find these
    practices super distracting when I started, yet
    by going into them time and time again, I find
    that I can maintain focus for longer and longer
    periods. This will be true for you, too, with
    regular practice.)

Practice this for ideally 5–10 minutes in the morning
to start your day, at the end of the day before you go to
bed, or at both times. Even a little bit is better than nothing, but a few full minutes at least is necessary to start
to untether you from your sense distractions and make
contact with the boundless, incredible energy that is
inside of you.

When you are done, sit for a moment in gratitude, and
watch for any realizations or ideas to rise up from inside
of you. Maybe you get some, maybe you don't, but either
way you should feel calmer than when you started. Just
keep observing!

Chapter 5

YOU ARE LOVE

"My Heavenly Father is love, and I am made in His image. I am the sphere of love in which all planets, all stars, all beings, all creation are glimmering. I am the love that pervades the whole universe."

— PARAMAHANSA YOGANANDA[1]

REAL LOVE

My whole relationship to love changed after I held my mother in my arms as she left her body.

We had discovered Mom had cancer on Valentine's Day 2017, much to our shock, because she had seemed her normal energetic self until that point. My first son, Emerson, turned one year old on March 26, that year. And then three days later, Mom passed, just six weeks after her first diagnosis. Everything moved so quickly that I still have trouble believing she is gone.

There was an extraordinary period between the hours of 1 and 3 A.M. right before she passed away. My mother, Sally, could no longer speak. But I asked her to squeeze my hand if she could still hear me. And squeeze she did. For two precious hours, her beautiful, big black eyes opened wide with love and a deep peace I had never before felt from her. I, on the other hand, bawled. And through my sobbing I poured my heart out. I kept saying over and over again, "Love never dies. I will love you forever!"

Then came the hard part. The really hard part. I could feel that she was clinging to life because she wanted to be there for my dad. They had been together for over 40 years, and they were inseparable. As I held her hand, I said, "Mom, it's okay to let go. I will take care of Daddy. I promise." I curled up in the hospital bed with her and wrapped my arms around her as I felt her breath slow. Then she let go and her spirit transcended.

One of the greatest gifts of my life was being right there with her, holding her as she transitioned. In the midst of my own pain, there was incredible beauty and freedom. Freedom for her. Freedom for True Love to emerge.

It was then I experienced the real truth of Yogananda's teaching: "Love gives without expecting anything in return."[2] When I told my mom to rest, it meant I would no longer be able to get love from her, at least not in the same way. I wouldn't be able to call her on the phone to say hi or to have her comfort me during times of stress or disappointment. She was not going to be there to hold my baby as he grew, to watch him walk. She wouldn't be there for holidays or for laughs or even tears. She simply was never going to be physically present in my life any longer.

I realized in those moments before she passed that I had to let go too. As tough as it was, I did. This mutual letting go transformed me and blew my heart wide open. Now, a few years later, I realized that my mom had given me the greatest gift of all. She allowed me to see that all of us, regardless of what we look like, our perceived limitations, or how we live, are a pure embodiment of love. My mom was love. You are love. I am love. Love is inside all the time.

When you start to get this, you will experience explosions of love that come from inside of you, for no particular reason, and they will start to occur more frequently.

LOVE IS WITHIN

In the *Self-Realization Fellowship Lessons*, Yogananda describes the often-tragic phenomenon of the Himalayan musk deer. The animal's aromatic musk scent is located in a sac beneath its abdominal skin. As the deer matures, it gets excited by the musk scent and desperately starts looking for its source. It sniffs under rocks, around trees, in flowers, searching everywhere it possibly can.

Finally, after a few weeks of seemingly fruitless searching, these deer grow increasingly restless and angry. Some of them stir themselves up into such a frenzy that they literally jump off high cliffs and fall to their deaths in the valleys below. All the while, the thing they were looking for—the source of the musk—was coming right from them. They never realized that what they were seeking was inside all along.

This is the way that most of us go about our search for love. We think it has to come from outside of us. We think it's going to come from our significant other, from our family members. Some of us seek fame and the adoration of fans (just think of social media).

But really, you don't "get" love from others. It's just that some people prompt you to feel the love that is already there in you. None of those external things are the source of love. In the best of times, they may be reflections of love, but a reflection is just that—an image. An image can provide so much to us—it might give us direction, reveal something hidden, but love transcends all images. Love is not a noun. It's not a thing. Love is a verb. It is that action that makes babies and flowers grow.

Love is the True Self in action.

ACCESSING TRUE LOVE

When we try to *get* love from outside of ourselves, attachments arise. We all want love, since it is our true nature, and feeling love is an inherent need that longs to be filled, sometimes to the point of desperation. We might make decisions that move us very far away from our authentic selves. This may include staying in a relationship for security because you are afraid of being alone, overly valuing your body as your source of worth to try to attract a mate, continuing to give lots of your energy to a friendship you have outgrown, or not really being yourself to try to please your parents.

All of this just feels so arduous! And yet love isn't actually tricky and difficult. Yogananda says love is very simple. Love is all about connecting with the True Self, the fountainhead of all love. "The greatest love you can experience is in communion with God in meditation,"[3] he teaches us. And that is essentially what this book is all about, namely, that through meditation, through our practice, we can experience the enlightenment, the freedom of peace and love that is our true identity. So yes, it's absolutely worth the effort to sit still and quiet the mind! For as Yogananda goes on to say, "When you meditate, love grows."[4]

We can know love is growing in our lives from internal markers. These markers include feeling more joy, patience, kindness, compassion, and connection to ourselves and to others all around us. External markers, such as how many fans or followers you have, how many people think you're hot, and how high you climb up in your field will never be the true indication of love. Love doesn't keep score. Love is not selfish. Love is always patient. Love is always calm.

ONENESS

You may have heard that everything is either love or fear. How does fear show up in our lives? It shows up as division and separation. The Sanskrit word for "delusion" is *maya*, and it is the force that divides, differentiates, and disharmonizes.[5] In real life, this looks like me versus you. Us versus them. Fear is the basis of feeling competitive with one another over appearance, feeling there's not enough success, time, resources, or anything else. This disconnection often manifests in depression and anxiety.

We do not have to choose fear. We do not have to buy into the delusion of separation, even as the news and the rest of the world tells us that's the way it is. We can feel with our own intuition that harmony, which is characterized by inclusivity not exclusivity, is the truth. Love is inclusive, so inclusive that *everyone* is included in it. Including every little baby and every single person that is alive and breathing! That is what Oneness means—that we are in a giant circle all together, and what happens to one person in this circle happens to the other. It is our job to keep looking out for one another.

At the core, we are all connected through Spirit, which pulses through each of us. The surface differences continue to become more and more trivial as we connect to the truth of love inside of each person. We are all different expressions, but ultimately have the same core. "Every reflection of love comes from the one Cosmic Love,"[6] says Yogananda.

For sure, there are going to be people we don't vibe with. We might not agree with people's values, their political opinions, the way they raise their kids. But underneath all of those seeming divisions, there is still a unifying principle. Everyone is still part of Oneness. Everyone is still ultimately love. Even that rotten sourpuss neighbor who always complains about your parking. Even that in-law or cousin who drives you crazy. We are all love.

Now, that doesn't mean we act like love all the time. Let's be real. Buddha and Jesus may have been able to embrace everyone fully, but that's a lot to ask of any of us! We're on the path but not quite there. Let's embrace instead where we are, be curious, and explore any aversion we might have toward others, whether it's people we know personally, politicians, celebrities, or whoever. In practical terms, Yogananda teaches us that while we might find that some people's behavior may be "ugly," we should try to focus on their positive traits. We don't have to ask them to join our softball team or go for a hike, but we don't have to tear them down either. Yogananda says that the path to really and truly feeling Omnipresent Love is to ultimately find it within every soul.

Self-Reflection

Who do you feel disconnected from? It could be an individual or a whole group of people. While you may not agree with the way they live their lives, can you see deep, deep down to who they really are? Even beyond the reactive, fearful behaviors, like those exhibited in the obnoxious attention-seekers, or the racist bigot, or the sexist narcissist at your work, what do you see underneath it all? Can you find a way to feel unity with them on some level, and drop the division? That's a tall order, I know, but imagine for 30 seconds that you could see past the super challenging behaviors. How do you feel? What do you feel?

GIVING LOVE TO BE LOVE

Now, when I say love is inside of us, that doesn't mean it can't exist outside of us as well. There are nearly 8 billion people in the world, and love exists in all of them as well, even though it may be hard for us to see sometimes. Day in and day out, many, if not most people, in the world are giving love to someone through kindness, charity, compassion, and forgiveness. The act of love allows us to *be* love, which, besides meditation, is the primary way that we can grow the love in our lives. This is probably why people feel so good volunteering or when they are helping to make the world a better place.

While love can be a hard thing to measure, the London School of Economics took a stab at it. They studied volunteering and found that the more people volunteered, the happier they were. They also built empathy, strengthened social bonds, and smiled more—all factors believed to increase the feelings of love.[7] This makes me think of a famous quote from Muhammad Ali: "Service to others is the rent you pay for your room here on earth."

Love is active; love is an action. Love can be a reaction too. Something you use when someone is a total jerk.

You are love because you have been loved and have been created by *love*. This is your inheritance, to know that Spirit is love and you are love and you are one with Spirit, with the True Self.

What does this mean in practical terms? Stop worrying about yourself. Do something for someone else. Help that person succeed. Don't be a doormat, but don't be afraid to be inconvenienced. Love is the only thing that, when given, comes back twofold. If I share an apple with you, I have only half an apple to eat. If I share my 10 dollars with you, I may have only 5 left. If I share love with you, what happens? Love doubles. Love is increased. Ultimately, love creates.

And if you want to find love, maybe put the dating apps aside for a while and do something good for another person. Go within and start to know yourself through meditation. I guarantee you will meet someone who is on the same wavelength. Once you give yourself away, you get yourself even more.

Self-Reflection: The Source of Love

The path to embodying true self-love is a journey. Reflections like this start to ignite realizations that can help the path forward, but they are certainly not going to get us to an "end" of the journey in a day. Keep reflecting and meditating, and your self-love will start to grow in its own pattern and time frame, like a beautiful lotus flower rising up out of the mud.

Take the time to reflect deeply, and write out in your journal the answers to the following questions:

1. Love is an action. What are the ways you've acted in love lately?

2. What is your relationship to validation or seeking love from others or outside of yourself?

3. What are ways that you may have been trying to "get" love that don't feel good to you anymore?

4. Say to yourself, "My True Self is love." What came up for you when you said that? Just observe and notice; don't judge.

RELATIONSHIP LOVE

We can't talk about love and not also talk about relationships, right? The right relationships can elevate your life. But relationships still don't replace the all-important, all-pervading self-love inside of you.

First, let's talk about romantic love. Have you ever been obsessed with finding a relationship when you were single? Thinking that once you found that one perfect partner it was going to fix the gnawing hole inside of you? The feeling of loneliness? Or have you ever stayed with someone because you wanted to be loved and paid attention to, even if it wasn't the right relationship?

Remember first and foremost to focus on connecting with yourself, in reflection, stillness, and meditation. Get to really know yourself, which is the precursor to self-love. When you do that first, you radiate a very powerful kind of energy out into the world. It's a highly attractive frequency. You become a person who emanates love rather than seeking it, and that will draw more potential partners to you than you could ever want!

And in all relationships, including your friendships and family, keep your focus on expansive Oneness love. For if you start to narrow your love, possessiveness, jealousy, or attachment can start to creep in. Yogananda tells us, "Attachment spoils family love, and all forms of human relationships, because it excludes others and is blindly possessive."[8] Jealousy is rooted in fear, which we know is the antithesis of love. It's divisive and destroys harmony. Successful relationships must have a strong foundation of trust. We trust our partners if we choose to stay with them; otherwise, we shouldn't stay. And we trust that we are connected to our children even as they grow and become independent of us. Love is not attachment, and we have to let go in *all* our relationships. That doesn't mean kicking your family to the curb, but it does mean willing the best in all circumstances.

Yogananda also talks about how important it is in friendships and all kinds of relationships to really and truly respect each other, and that means "The acceptance of each one's individuality—two souls, different in character, pulling together the chariot of life to a common goal. Truth must be the standard upon which a relationship is based."[9]

FORGIVENESS: PATH TO OPENING LOVE

Forgiveness is a powerful way to access more love in everything we do. There are so many occurrences in life, from our early infanthood and childhood on, that can leave us with little and perhaps not-so-little wounds. These wounds, if not allowed to heal properly, become scars that block the flow of love. These little wounds keep us reacting in the same way, upset about the same things, ruminating about the same past stuff over and over again. It's not only a tremendous waste of energy, but it dams up the streams of love that are meant to flow in a million different ways throughout our entire lives.

The only way to open these blockages is through forgiveness. This involves letting go of the hurt and allowing it to flow away from you. This can be a difficult process, but it is something that can revolutionize our lives.

Science agrees that forgiveness even benefits our health. A study on the physiological effects of forgiveness published in *Psychological Science* theorized that forgiveness "may free the wounded person from a prison of hurt and vengeful emotion, yielding both emotional and physical benefits, including reduced stress, less negative emotions, fewer cardiovascular problems, and improved immune system performance."[10] This study even found that we can look differently when we don't forgive! Physiological measurements showed that during "unforgiveness," participants showed greater corrugator EMG activity, a measure of tension in the brow area of the face, which we all know leads to wrinkles!

Sometimes it's easy to hold on to hurts. Our egos tell us that we had no right to be treated a certain way, that we were wronged. The ego isn't necessarily wrong, but just like holding on to food inside your digestive system can cause blockages, holding on to pain can lead to mental, spiritual, and emotional obstructions as well. And to be perfectly straight, when we hold on to pain—to the wrongs someone has done to us—we are also holding that experience over another's head. And that can give us a false sense of power. It's a form of revenge—often passive-aggressive revenge, but revenge nonetheless. In the end, we are the ones who get burned by this desire for retribution.

It can also lead to skewed righteousness or the feeling that you are better than another. Forgiveness is like taking a spiritual laxative—you don't want to hold on to all that crap, so get rid of it. Let it go.

When you do decide to forgive, you will feel a weight lifted. The weight being lifted is actually the release of a block of love. Ever hold a block of anything? Ice? Wood? Stone? Blocks are heavy! Forgiveness is an energetic release, akin to rubbing out a big muscle knot. When you feel the freedom of forgiveness once, you will find it easier to let go over and over again.

One of the most important acts of forgiveness is to forgive yourself. We've all screwed up in different ways. Think of the time you might have yelled at your parents when you were really frustrated with yourself, botched a project and got disciplined for it, told a lie or talked non-sense about someone and it got back to them. Instead of continuing to beat yourself up over a past mistake or indiscretion, move toward an experience of self-compassion. Today, you are not the same person you were a year ago, last month, or even yesterday. We are all growing—granted at different rates—but we still grow.

Think about it. If you knew then what you know now, would you have treated your roommate that way, would you have walked away from someone you cared about, would you have gossiped behind someone's back? Probably not. Your path continues to unfold, just as everyone else's does. You weren't "bad." It's just that your level of understanding was limited at the time.

As we step into more alignment with love, we find that we feel more Oneness within ourselves and more Oneness around us. We find that we have the love inside of us, and we are the ones we've been seeking for love all along.

Self-Reflection: Forgiveness Practice

I've done different versions of forgiveness practices, and they have significantly made me feel lighter and happier in my day-to-day life. Who among us doesn't harbor at least some resentment toward one or both of our parents, colleagues, friends, ex-partners, teachers, and so on? Resentment weighs us down, and it's like stagnant, stuck energy, not dissimilar to the physical blockages and toxins that can accrue in our G.I. tracts.

Forgiveness is a tricky thing, and it's certainly not easy. We can forgive someone who has hurt us, but that doesn't mean we are condoning someone's bad behavior. And forgiveness takes time. If you break a bone, it can take a few weeks to *start* healing. You may get your cast removed, but you will still experience some pain and need physical therapy, often for long periods of time. The same goes for physical, emotional, and psychological injuries that someone might inflict on us.

Forgiveness takes time, and this exercise will allow you to take the rehabilitating steps necessary to heal. And this involves transforming hurt, bitterness, anger, sadness, or trauma into a lightness of being. This is for *your* freedom, your unfolding path to enlightenment and freedom. Do this for yourself, not anyone else.

This is a version of a practice inspired by one that I worked with at a neurofeedback training that I did, which I wanted to share with you because I found it highly effective.[11] I hope it helps you, too, to lighten your energy and any kind of anger or resentment you are still carrying in your body.

1. First, take a seat in a quiet place and ideally meditate for at least a few minutes. This is important to help regulate your thinking and help you access the feelings in your body.

2. Now recall a specific event with someone who caused you pain and suffering.

3. Feel the event in your body. Be specific. This event could manifest as a sensation in your neck and throat, in your heart, belly, or somewhere else. Really feel the sensations in order to process them. Don't keep thinking about the event at all; just focus completely on your body and the sensations that are arising. Don't rush this part—wait until all big sensations and feelings have subsided before you go on to the next step.

4. Next, focus on finding something positive from what happened. It could be that you got stronger, more self-reliant, or maybe that you simply learned how to deeply forgive. Allow the feeling of gratitude to flood through your body.

5. Try to see the situation from the other person's perspective. Try to understand why they did what they did. Maybe this person was hurt or came from an ultra-wounded place, maybe he or she was having a particularly bad day, or maybe he or she simply had limited understanding at the time. Try to bring empathy and compassion in here, which, along with the processing and gratitude of the prior steps, are some of the most powerful healing energies you can bring in. Remember, this is for your own healing!

6. Finally, close with love. You can bring your hands together in prayer, or Anjali mudra, decide to let go, and bless the situation with love. Bring love to all the people involved (if you can do this, it's a sign that you've really forgiven!), including yourself, and close with surrender to the great healing and transformative power of love.

Other Practical Ways to Feel More Love in Your Life

1. **Replace judgment with compassion.** The more we can see our own wounds, the more we realize that other people have them too. And that they aren't necessarily "bad," but they come from a place of limited perspective. They are experiencing blockages of love too. When you look at a situation with compassion, you can transform it, and in the process help others to rethink their behaviors and actions.

2. **Be grateful.** Gratitude allows you to shift your focus into positivity and goodness, and ultimately love. When you focus on lack, that's what you get in life. Lack sucks. If you lack water long enough, you will die. If you lack food long enough, you will die. If you lack love long enough, you will die. Instead, tap into plenty. When you focus on abundance, you get that in life too. You realize that there is so much in your life already, and when you are appreciative, more comes to you. Moreover, according to Harvard Health Publishing, psychology research shows that gratitude helps people feel more positive emotions, improve their health, and build stronger relationships.[12]

3. **Bring love to your day-to-day interactions.** It's the small, daily steps that make a difference, and I would also extend that to interactions in your day—people you come across in the coffee shop or post office, the people you pass in the gym or elevators. Bring love to these

interactions and see how it grows across your whole life.

4. **Have only love in your heart for others.**
   Yogananda teaches us that "The way to make people good is to see the good in them."[13] When you really see through the surface and the behaviors into people's hearts, and you focus on those positive qualities, it's amazing that they can start to embody more of those qualities, at least in relation to you. What you focus on tends to expand, as we discussed earlier, so focus on the love inside of others, and see how your relationships transform and how it becomes easier to get along with others.

Chapter 6

YOU ARE WHOLE

"Is a diamond less valuable because it is covered with mud? God sees the changeless beauty of our souls. He knows we are not our mistakes."

— PARAMAHANSA YOGANANDA[1]

THE BIG PART OF YOU

What does "you are whole" mean? At first, you might be reminded of the current, more mainstream movement toward eating whole, unprocessed foods (thankfully!). Yet it also refers to something much larger.

Many of us tend to focus on the surface stuff that we can see, such as our appearance, the labels we put on ourselves (woman, man, mother, father, wife, librarian, accountant, lawyer, young, middle-aged, student, and so on), the things we've done, the accomplishments we are still chasing. Yet all of that is actually tiny compared to what's underneath. Underneath what author Wayne Dyer calls "that one percent of living life through our physical form" is something so much bigger, namely the True Self.[2]

You can tinker with the surface stuff all you like! Some of it's fun, and some of it's not so fun. But if you don't connect with the part of you that is whole, then you will continue to feel small, no matter what, and that translates to feeling lack. As we already discussed, lack is a block to confidence, self-love, and peace. And "lack energy" repels love, beautiful relationships, and opportunities. It is the opposite of whole, and as Yogananda teaches us, "Unless a wave dissolves itself and becomes one with the ocean, it remains inordinately limited."[3]

Once you can tap into that wholeness, your entire relationship to life will change. You open up the pathway for all sorts of new and exciting relationships to come into your life, as well as opportunities that reflect your growing self-awareness, abundance, love, and ultimately the freedom that is enlightenment.

WHEN YOUR BEHAVIOR ISN'T WHO YOU ARE

All of us desire to be the best possible person we can be. Many times, we fall flat. We act in angry, mean, and resentful ways when we feel slighted or misunderstood. We can react from the wounded places inside of us, and then we feel guilty for our behavior. It's important to learn lessons from our life experiences and then move on. Yogananda teaches us, "Cultivate forgetfulness of past wrong and vengeful feelings, and encourage only the remembrance of good."[4] He goes on to say, "Remembering only the good experiences of the past, you shall eventually remember your oneness with Spirit."[5]

The issue is when we do the opposite, and we keep fixating on all the "bad" stuff we've done. The guilt drags on, which is dangerous because holding on to long-term guilt can lead to shame.

Shame is a heavy kind of self-judgment and arises when part of one's self is perceived to be inadequate, inappropriate, or immoral.[6] But really, the whole experience of your past only exists in this now moment as thoughts. When you really think about it, it's actually pretty preposterous that we continue to allow ourselves to feel bad and shameful about our own thoughts!

Shame is strongly linked to depression, as evidenced in one large-scale meta-analysis in which researchers examined 108 studies involving more than 22,000 subjects.[7] Other researchers have also found a connection between shame and anxiety.[8] Research has even found detrimental physical health consequences related to shame, including the release of the steroid hormone cortisol[9] and proinflammatory cytokines (PIC)[10] linked to reducing our immunity and wearing down our body's health in general.

When we start identifying those behaviors and characteristics as who we are, we move very far away from our true nature. We start to think less of ourselves. That we're no good, that we can't be loved, that we're not worth the time of others. This belief system is a bunch of BS.

First of all, you and I are on the journey to enlightenment, so none of us are perfect. We make mistakes and learn, and sometimes we make the same mistake a few times, and then we learn. So it goes. And secondly, while your True Self is always shining through, your surface behaviors are all just parts of your humanness. Part of your ego trying to protect itself from perceived dangers, for instance, rejection. None of those qualities are the real you. It's the hurt, scared, fearful part of you trying to take over and project its pain. Yogananda calls the ego the *pseudosoul*, the shadow of the soul. So stop obsessing! A lot of us may think we need to somehow repay what we've done in the form of beating ourselves up and feeling guilty indefinitely. This kind of thinking has to stop.

Think of the ego as a pain-in-the-ass teenager. They think they know everything, but deep down they don't have a clue and they know it. Challenge teenagers on a belief, and what do they do? They often go on the attack and hurl insults your way, along with illogical, stubborn behavior. I know. I was a teenager once. So were you! This can be unsettling and downright debilitating. But in the end, the tirade isn't coming from a place of superiority, but from a place of uncertainty and fear.

That being said, the ego isn't bad, just misguided.

KEEP MOVING FORWARD

As we continue to journey toward living life from the True Self and continue with our meditations and practice, we embody more of the high-vibration qualities associated with enlightenment: love, peace, joy. And those qualities are in alignment with who we really are. Tapping into the flow of authenticity will continue to outwardly influence more and more of your actions.

My friend, who I will call Alyssa, whom I met at a women's circle (more on this in just a moment), went through a rough phase where she felt lonely and lost touch with her own strength and voice. She was feeling increasingly distant from her husband, who still wanted to party every weekend, while she was continually gravitating toward a quieter life. She started spending time with a man she met at her gym, who was giving her a lot of attention. One thing led to another, and she had an affair. She felt terrible and incredibly shameful over the incident, and really tortured herself about it. She came clean about the incident to her husband and apologized to him.

Nevertheless, the marriage ended in divorce—and a lot of drama. Her then ex-husband e-mailed their entire wedding list of 270 people, including the grandmothers and lifelong family friends, and told them what had happened. In the midst of all the drama, Alyssa also got fired from her job.

You can imagine that Alyssa hit rock bottom. She had no job, no friends, and no money. Her parents were furious with her, and she was attacked so much on social media that she deleted all her accounts.

Alyssa harbored so much shame over the incident that she gained 15 pounds, and the next two people she dated were incredibly stingy with her and also cheated on her. Soon thereafter, she hit her second rock bottom. She realized that all the guilt she was holding on to was still manifesting in her world around her and was affecting what she was attracting. Through a lot of journaling, meditating, and connecting with a new community she met at the women's circles, she finally forgave herself, a full three years after the incident. Today she is much lighter and happier. She has accepted herself, and even her body, for the first real time. She is also consciously single, allowing herself the space to get to really know herself in a deep way.

I'm not saying there is ever a justification to cheat or be dishonest in any way. But I am saying that we've all done things of various degrees that we aren't exactly proud of. Should that define who we are for the rest of our lives? Are we supposed to wear a big scarlet letter stamped on our forehead, in this case a big *C* for cheater or a big *G* for gossip or *L* for liar or whatever? Where's the line between bearing our lesson and letting it go?

MEETING EACH OTHER WHERE WE ARE

One of the reasons why there are so many problems in the world is that we have trouble meeting people where they are. We have expectations of what others should be instead of just letting them be.

Yogic philosophy teaches us the path of nonduality. This means we just *are*. No judgment. Nonduality means that you will have many different aspects of yourself rise and fall, like waves, but underneath it all, you are still you. The deep-down essence of you has *always* been there. Even through all your behaviors.

And believe me, I have acted in ways that are judgmental, mean, and petty, but after spending so much time with Yogananda's teachings and getting in touch with the True Self, I've let go of a lot of these behaviors, which are really all mirrors of acting from the wounded ego.

The esteemed Swami Sri Yukteswar, the guru of Yogananda, says, "Forget the past. The vanished lives of all men [and women] are dark with many shames. Human conduct is ever unreliable until man is anchored in the Divine. Everything in future will improve if you are making a spiritual effort now."[11] So don't let your past hamper your progress now and going forward. *Choose* to learn from it, to integrate the lessons to help inform better choices and decisions going forward, and to let yourself move on.

You, me, and everyone we meet is exactly where they are on their journey. When we can meet others where they are and look them in the eye and really see them underneath their moods and behavior, that is when you know that you are making progress. Further, you are moving closer to being compassionate with yourself.

Self-Reflection: Identifying with the Light

Since we've been talking about the True Self a lot, which might be a brand-new concept to you, I want to give you a visual to go along with it.

Imagine a beam of white light that shines down through the center of you, like your spine does. But instead of tuning in to the physicality of vertebrae and nerves, imagine that this bright white light represents you at your core as pure energy. It beams down like a spotlight through the entirety of your being.

When you move around the world, when you think about yourself and your true identity, you can tune in to the True Self by visualizing and identifying with that brilliant, all-perfect shining light inside of you. You can also start to see people for who they really are by focusing on seeing the light inside of them, even if it's temporarily hidden underneath some pretty immature or annoying behaviors.

The light is the True Self, and it is the Divinity inside of each of us. Now, it doesn't mean that you have to trample down on the humanness within you, the struggling human who stumbles along in life and messes up. But it also means that you put things in the proper order: your Divine side is already perfect and whole, and you recognize that it's your true identity. Yet at the same time you love and feel compassion for the humanness in you that is in the process of becoming your fullest truth. We accept her, forgive her, and love her as she makes her way back to fully merging with the True Self along the often-messy journey of life, which is full of ups, downs, and lots of lessons.

YOU ARE THE SUN AND THE MOON

A few years ago, I began attending women's circles, which is essentially when a group of women gather and share what is present for them and what is going on in their lives. Advice is not given (unless it's specifically asked for). Rather, it's about simply holding space for one another. The circle is a safe place for vulnerability and allows each woman to stand in her truth and be witnessed.

The vulnerability part felt pretty radical to me when I started. I wasn't used to sitting around and speaking up so openly in front of others. Yet I immediately understood what an immensely healing tool this kind of tribal community connection can be. These communities are often a missing link in one's total wellness journey to feeling whole.

I got super into women's circles, and soon started to lead my own. I then went on to create an entire virtual Solluna Circle program. (Come join us! You'll find info on my website.) Something amazing, magical, and mystical happens in the circle. Sometimes tears are shed, sometimes not. But just by being there, by listening intently and being honest and vulnerable about struggles and what is really happening in our lives, transformation happens. We are mirrors to each other.

It is powerful to take off your mask, so to speak, and just really and truly be yourself. We wear masks in so many ways to so many people in our lives: our co-workers, our social media followers, even our friends. But in the circle no mask is needed, and so the deep healing can come from really and truly being seen as yourself.

Many of the women in the circles reported a tremendous relief from being able to share what was in their hearts. And many also remarked on the shifts in their lives that they were able to implement from the sharing that went on in the circles.

The following activity is a way to have your own personal circle with yourself. It's a sacred, private space of self-reflection that can actually move a lot of repressed energy that comes from disowning parts of ourselves. This requires vulnerability, because you may have protected yourself against seeing these things with a hard, turtle-like shell of unawareness. Rejecting any part of ourselves is self-denial. Rejection is stagnancy and repression. When we allow our wholeness to bloom, we can become fully alive and fully passionate. And we can then truly begin to love ourselves. Not in a surface, temporary way. But in the real way.

The more you can see, the more you can let go and the more you will be living from the place of the True Self. Then you claim more of *you*—the love, the beauty, the lightness, the joy that you have been keeping away from yourself.

Self-Reflection: *You* Are the Sun and the Moon

In your journal, open to a new page and draw a vertical line down the middle. To the left, draw a sun and write "I Am the Sun" at the very top. Though it's not as linear as this, we are going to use the sun symbol for your "positive" traits. List the traits you like about yourself. Kind, compassionate, good friend, and so on might be some words in there.

Now, to the right of the vertical line, draw a moon and write "I Am the Moon" at the top of the page. Make a list of traits that are part of your shadow, the parts that you do not like to identify within yourself but that deep down, you know that you exhibit at times. This list is a little harder to make, right? It can feel tough to write some of these down, but remember that great power comes with awareness. Don't hold back. Qualities like impatient, mean, jealous, lazy, and angry might be on your list. Do not distract yourself during this process (which might be an easy temptation). Don't start scrolling on your phone or picking at your nails! Let all the words come out.

Here is an example of what a list may look like:

I Am the Sun	I Am the Moon
Loving	Judgmental
Kind	Cheap/Stingy
Reliable	Envious
Patient	Impatient
Open-minded	Closed-minded
Organized	Fearful
Thoughtful	Careless
Good listener	Bad listener
Inclusive	Exclusive
Warm	Standoffish
Compassionate	Bitchy
Charismatic	Stubborn
Forgiving	Greedy
Generous	Selfish

When you are done, compare your two lists. Take some deep belly breaths and let yourself sit in the absolute fullness of you, all the parts. Let whatever feelings and self-judgments rise and fall. **Remind yourself that these qualities are ultimately attached to surface behaviors that are parts of your ego; they are not the real you. The True Self is beyond all of those qualities. The True Self just is.** But going through the process of seeing and acknowledging all your behaviors and tendencies fully is part of the process of integrating them into your wholeness. It's part of embodying your own "sun-moon" cycle.

Let this process take as long as it does, but please focus on it for at least ten or more minutes. When it is complete, close your eyes and affirm the mantra "I am whole."

Besides hiding from general characteristics like being impatient or petty, we can hold on to the deep shame of past things we have done. Like Alyssa, who I mentioned earlier in the chapter, things that don't fit into the neat little labels we base our sense of self upon can make us feel guilty and shameful and bad about ourselves.

For example, I would not have thought of myself as someone who would get a divorce, have C-sections rather than natural births (although boy, did I try not to!), be a single mom, or be judgmental or snippy at times, but I have done all of these in my life. I definitely felt some shame around these things in the past that didn't fit in with my constructed outward identity until I was able to process them. Now I can talk about them openly and without shame, because of this practice and work. I own these parts of me, and they don't own me. It's so incredibly freeing.

It doesn't mean that we have to publicly advertise all that we've done like some kind of forced confession to the world. But what it does mean is that within yourself, you must work toward accepting all the things that you have done in the process of integration back into your wholeness. You are the one who knows all that's happened along the wild, beautiful, unpredictable, challenging journey of your life: the willing hook-ups with less-than-impressive guys when you were a bit tipsy, the gossiping, the cheating on a test (or on your partner), the times you could have been a better friend.

Yogananda says, "Avoid dwelling on all the wrong things you have done. They do not belong to you now. Let them be forgotten. It is attention that creates habit and memory."[12] So remember not to keep focusing on your past behaviors by giving them more and more *new* attention. **Rather, own all the qualities you show and have ever shown, and once you see them and allow them to be felt and accepted, you can be free of them. Take the lessons, let the rest go, and move forward, free and whole!**

YOU ARE BEYOND NUMBERS

Part of embodying wholeness as your true nature is not letting numbers completely define you. Sure, numbers can help give us some broad strokes in how we are doing, so I'm not suggesting we throw out all numbers and pretend they don't exist in the world. That would be delusional. Obey speed limits and pay attention to your blood pressure number. I am suggesting that we stop giving numbers all our power, whether it's the number of pounds or kilos you weigh or obsessing over your current salary or how many followers you have and so on. If these numbers can profoundly affect your mood or your self-worth, then it's time to put numbers back into their proper perspective.

And what's ironic about our society's obsession with losing weight is that I've always found that when we feel truly good and centered and connected to ourselves, we have a much easier time dropping unwanted weight without the fixation. Why is that? Because when we feel good, we have less stress, our digestion tends to function better, and we feel more naturally motivated to work out and eat healthier foods. We are less prone to give in to food cravings when we have a source for feeling joyful and connected to our natural energy from within through our meditations. Then we don't have to try to shift our energy from outside sources like food. So in the end, it's way more important—and effective—to continue to work on feeling in touch with the deeper, expansive energy of your True Self versus getting bogged down with numbers.

Yogananda cautions against becoming too preoccupied with numbers. For instance, he counsels us to keep our age private. Instead, we can affirm, "I am immortal." If you get too caught up in the year in which you were born, or in other words, your chronological age, you find that obsessing over it can create anxiety, which only wears you down. You may even start to mold yourself into what you "should" look like at a certain age. For example, someone in their 50s could start looking "old" because they have a picture in their mind of what a 50-year-old should look like: gray, hunched over, with a potbelly. Get rid of those ideas! The mind is powerful, and if we believe in the absolute power of numbers, they will have that absolute power over us.

Here's the truth: what's limitless and true can't be measured by numbers. Think of love. Can you measure love on a scale? Nope. Can you weigh wisdom? Or how about truth or true beauty? (We're definitely not talking about beauty pageant scores here.) No. By tuning in to limitlessness, your reality expands. It is not confined to arbitrary numbers.

Stay living in the limitless. We can't get enlightened if we think we are small. And in the end, numbers are pretty small beans.

WHOLENESS IN NATURE

Wholeness is found in nature. It is actually one of the defining qualities of nature, found in each blade of grass and rock that unapologetically stands as it is. The ocean is who she is and will ever be: stormy and slapping waves one day and serene another. The branch of the tree may be gnarled and bent, but she stands strong just as she is too.

The sun shines during the day, trading off with the darkness of night. It's not that one is the "good" or the "bad" part, but it's that it's all one complete cycle. Mother Nature *is* the light and the dark and the sunrise and the sunset, plus all the in-between parts.

She is all the forms, yet underneath it all is the pervasive energy of Spirit. And so it is with you. You are everything on the surface, and at the same time you are the wholeness of the True Self, shining through it all.

Self-Reflection:
Absorbing Wholeness from Nature

We can learn from immersion. And the unchanging wholeness found in nature is a good teacher to sit with.

For this exercise, simply find a spot in nature you are drawn to. It can be a park if you live in a city, or the edge of the ocean or lake, the mountains, your lawn, or a tree at your kids' playground.

Look around with unjudging, open eyes. Notice how everything in nature just *is*. Sit right on the earth (if possible) for at least 10–20 minutes with the being-ness of Mother Nature. Don't listen to music. Don't speak. Just be still, observe, and witness. Feel the power of wholeness of just being and not doing. If possible, do your meditation practice as outlined in Chapters 7, 10, and 20.

Practical Tips for Embodying Wholeness in Your Life

1. **Choose to release.** Choose a past action you regret. It could be losing your temper with your kid or your significant other, lying, being petty, stealing, or whatever. Recall the incident and let whatever feelings rise up in your body when you do so.

    Then take a deep breath and find the lesson(s) that you learned from the incident. It could be as simple as, "Well, I'm not going to do that again!" Close your eyes, place both of your hands over your heart, and say aloud or internally, "I now let it go." And mean it. As much as you can in the moment, feel that you've done all you can now, the past is the past as Yogananda says, and fully let it go. Let any feelings rise up and then subside.

    As you continue your meditation practice and journaling, you may become more and more self-aware of other incidents you are holding on to. Please repeat this exercise at any time for each incident to keep letting go of past behavior and instead focus on wholeness *now*.

2. **Shift your focus.** The less you focus on numbers, the less they will control you. Throw out your scale; stop checking out how many likes you got on your social media post every 10 seconds. Stop telling people how old you are in every conversation. Stop apologizing to yourself and those around you that you currently have X amount of money versus Y.

   The more anxious you are about numbers, the more you deplete yourself. It's like trading in the infinite center for the limiting finite. Would you ever trade unlimited abundance for a $100 bill? Probably not.

   Adopt an attitude of confidence. Keep your energy and your thoughts focused on your inner nature, which is limitless, and unbound by any numbers.

3. **Focus on how you feel.** Tune in to your body and how you feel in your clothes, and how *you* feel walking around in the world. Don't let the scale or the birth year on your birth certificate tell you how to feel. If you feel great, then keep going. If you feel bloated and have low energy, then do something about it to feel better. Either way, it's more powerful to attune to your body and inner feelings than to ignore them and rely on outside sources.

4. **Remember you are the core, not the shell.** Think of a coconut. Have you ever seen one freshly chopped from a tree? The outer shell is a few inches of thick, rough, and weathered

wood. That's not the essence of the coconut, though. Beneath the shell is the fruit: the snow-white meat and the sweet water. The deliciousness of life—that which sustains—comes from the inside. Always remember that.

Go to your core and live there. Don't identify with your shell, which is characterized by things you may have done in the past, your triggers and wounds, your weight, age, calorie count, height, current savings, and salary. It's not the real you. And by the way, as the mighty coconut teaches us, the core is *so* much more delicious!

Chapter 7

PRACTICE:
Meditation, PART I:
FOUNDATION

*"Many people unsuccessfully strive for a material
goal all their lives, failing to realize that if they had
put forth one-tenth of the concentration used in seeking
worldly things into an effort to find God first, they
could then have had fulfillments of not only
some, but all of their hearts' desires."*

— PARAMAHANSA YOGANANDA[1]

Ancient yogic wisdom teaches us that meditation is
the single most important practice that exists for enlightenment and personal transformation. Period. Not too
many things in life are this clear-cut, so it's nice to find a
real truth!

Over the last four decades, the modern world has taken
notice. There are now countless programs, classes, centers,
and apps on meditation. Which is the one to follow? There
isn't a right or wrong answer. But it is key, if your goal
is enlightenment, to follow a path that originates from a

realized master, or guru. The term *guru* is a pretty weighty word in Sanksrit. It literally means "one that leads you from darkness (*gu*) to light (*ru*)."

Just as you don't want to learn how to wire a house from someone who's never wired more than a school science experiment, you want to learn meditation from someone who knows what she or he is talking about. Someone who's been to the top of the enlightenment mountain and can show us a path to get there ourselves.

When I discovered Yogananda's teachings and meditation techniques, it was obvious that they were culled from great wisdom. Kriya Yoga comes from a lineage of great yoga teachers that dates back millennia. So Yogananda's meditation techniques are tried and true.

To me, learning from the path of a true guru is like creating the solid foundation for a container. Once you have a solid container, like a bowl, and you've plugged some of the leaks, like self-doubt and wasting energy by being overrun by fear, then you can start to fill the "bowl" of your life with what you want.

Secret, ancient yogic teachings all used to be passed down orally, directly from teacher to student. Yogananda was the first to write down the Kriya Yoga teachings and help make them more accessible to people everywhere, because he saw that the busy, confusing, modern world increasingly needed them.

A number of the practices and meditations I offer in this book are adapted from instruction given by Yogananda during his public talks and writings and made available in his published works. If you are drawn to going deeper, please check out Yogananda's *Self-Realization Fellowship Lessons*, information that you can find in the Resources section. These lessons go much deeper into the Kriya Yoga science. At the heart of Kriya Yoga are specific techniques that help to quiet both your body and mind, and make it possible to withdraw the energy and attention from the usual turbulence of thoughts, emotions, and sensory perceptions, enabling you to experience increasingly deeper inner peace and connection with the True Self.

In this section, we are going to create a solid foundation for meditation that you can build on as you progress further and further on your journey.

Let's get started.

Beginning Meditation Instructions

1. **First, choose a practice spot.**

    In a totally ideal world, you would meditate in the same place every day, as energy builds over time. When you practice in the same spot, it signals to your brain and body that it's your time to drop into the gap.

    Your meditation spot could be a little corner of your bedroom or your living room, or even a closet! You can have a special chair you use, or you can simply sit on a cushion. I have an altar and a meditation spot in the corner of my bedroom, which I use for my evening meditations, after my children are in bed. But in the morning, both kids are currently in my bed from sunrise or before and on, so the only way I can maintain my morning practice is to just sit up in bed with them and meditate. Right in the midst of nursing and playing around me!

    This is not ideal, and it won't be the way my morning practice is forever. But I bring this up to show that you, too, can create consistency in your practice even in the midst of your busy (sometimes crazy!) life. It may not be exactly perfect, but so long as you are consistent and putting out the effort, you are going to make progress and take steps forward. And the results will be *so* worth it all.

2. **Get into the proper position.**
    Yogananda says something along the lines that trying to meditate with a bent spine is like trying to shoot a bent arrow. Posture is important! We are working with the energy in your spine and brain, so details really matter here. Here are some things to focus on:
    Your two options for sitting are either (1) in a straight chair or (2) in a cross-legged position on the floor. For the latter, use a cushion to slightly elevate your hips, which can make it more comfortable to sit for longer periods.
    Lift your spine so that your shoulders are over your hips. Make sure your chin is parallel with the floor (not jutting down, which is our go-to posture in this world of incessant cell phone use).
    If you are sitting in a chair, don't let your back slump against the back of the chair. This constricts the energy that we are working to "magnetize" up and down your spine.
    Make any little adjustments when you first get into position—a little head shake, a few shoulder rolls, fidgeting around with your hips. Then let your body go. The goal is to create a comfortable position where you can feel stable

and yet relaxed. This helps you forget about your body as you go into your practice.

Of course, this will take time, as we all may feel a bit squirmy sitting at first. The body can be a huge distraction. You might get an itch, your leg might fall asleep, or while adjusting your posture you might give yourself a wedgie. Make sure all wedgies are cleared before meditation!

3. **Start with an intention.**

Intention is key in any endeavor, and this includes your meditations. Bring your hands together in Anjali mudra (or prayer position) and say your intention to yourself. Choose something that personally resonates. It can be simple and basic, or more involved. Whatever suits you. Here are some examples of intentions:

I am Peace. I am Love.

I am present now.

I am calm and focused.

I am the True Self.

Spirit, you and I are One. Help me feel our connection.

God, help me to awaken your love in my heart. And may I help awaken your love in all hearts I encounter.

A Preliminary Breathing Exercise
by Paramahansa Yogananda [2]

"When you are established in the meditation pose just described, the next preparation for meditation is to rid the lungs of accumulated carbon dioxide, which causes restlessness.

"Expel the breath through the mouth in a double exhalation: 'huh, huhhh.' (This sound is made with the breath only, not the voice.)

"Then inhale deeply through the nostrils and tense the whole body to a count of six.

"Expel the breath through the mouth in a double exhalation, 'huh, huhhh' and relax the tension.

"Repeat this three times."

4. **Breathe and watch the gaps.**

   You can see how we are building our foundation from the previous exercises we've practiced. After doing the breathing exercise, spend some time just watching your breath as you sit quietly. Ideally this would be at least 5–10 minutes, as you are getting started with your practice. Here are some key reminders of this technique:

   As I mentioned in Chapter 4, pay attention to the gaps, the spaces *between* your inhales and exhales, where your breath takes a natural pause. As you pay attention to your breath, it will start to naturally slow down, and the gaps between inhales and exhales will start to expand. Do not try to force your breath to be any certain kind of pattern or count. Simply watch it and be calm.

5. **Close in gratitude.**

    When you've completed your practice, bring your hands together in prayer position in front of your heart. Take a moment to be grateful for your breath and your practice, and whatever else spontaneously arises from your heart. You can also say a prayer if that resonates with you here.

    We will continue to build on the practice in the upcoming sections. Of this Yogananda was emphatic: dedicate time each day to meditation wherein you can attune yourself with your True Self. Consistency is key. Make them part of your life, and part of your day!

A few more practical notes:

1. Put your phone in airplane mode to cut back on distractions.

2. Try to always do your meditation practice on an empty stomach.

3. Strive for at least 10 minutes to spend in your practice in the morning, ideally first thing before you get on your phone or eat or do any calls. Of course, spend as much time as possible in your practice. Go longer if you have the time!

4. Strive to also do your practice in the evenings if possible, for at least 10 minutes, before dinner or

before bed. As noted above, stay in your practice longer if possible. If you can't do the full time, even a few minutes to stay consistent is good.

5. Don't get frustrated when thoughts intrude while you're meditating. The more you practice, the more your mind will begin to slow down and the greater the gaps will be between thoughts. Getting your mind under control is definitely going to take practice. Think of how long it's been allowed to run rampant. It's like a wild horse that needs to be tamed. Be patient and keep bringing your mind back to center by focusing on your breath every time it wanders (which may be a lot at first!).

PART II

Chapter 8

YOU ARE PEACE

"Retire to the center of your being, which is calmness."

— PARAMAHANSA YOGANANDA[1]

IN THE TORNADO OF LIFE

Sometimes I feel like I have the same attention span as my five-year-old, running in one direction and making a mess, then running in another direction before cleaning it up. I might half finish an e-mail before getting up to clean up my son Emerson's spilled smoothie, only to then notice Moses, the baby, is wailing. It's at these times I start my "mom jig," as I call it, the endless rocking dance to try to get him to settle down. In the middle of all of this, I might remember to text someone on my team to reach out to a great potential podcast guest who popped into my head. By the time I get back to my computer, I've completely forgotten what I was trying to say in that e-mail in the first place.

So many of us live busy, chaotic lives, and inside we are a bundle of restless energies. We often feel confused and worried. These responses to our responsibilities make daily life so much harder! I know that when I get overly stressed, I can pick arguments about nothing. I guess my stress needs to go somewhere, so I sometimes project it onto innocent bystanders, who, sadly, are often loved ones. Then I feel guilty and expend a lot of emotional energy to fix the situations I cause. Though I've gotten way better over the years, there are times when disorder inside of me manifests as disorder outside of me.

And yet we all have within us the capacity for stillness and equanimity. Yogananda called this "calmness" and taught at length about the importance of maintaining a healthy and stable nervous system, which is the bridge connecting our bodies to the outside world around us.

Our nervous system has a lot to maintain, including helping to regulate our endocrine system, which controls our hormones. Our nervous system also has the big job of maintaining homeostasis, or equilibrium, in our bodies. While our bodies and minds may have been built to withstand wild swings in our health and in the outside environment, they are always trying to return to a place of peace. That's why a half hour after running a marathon (or six minutes, if you're really fit like my friend, triathlete Brendan Brazier), a runner's heart will return to a steady, even beat, even though it had been beating a mile a minute just a short time before.

Nowadays, the adverse effects of stress on our bodies have been well documented in thousands of research papers. Stress responses on our body can range from altering our heart rate and our ability to digest properly to triggering contributing factors that lead to disease and pathological conditions.[2] Moreover, stress can also wear down our mental health, contributing to depression and anxiety.[3] It's no wonder that the researchers recognize stress as the number one proxy killer disease today.[4]

Yogananda gives the analogy of a calm lake. It is a pure, reflective mirror. But if you throw a rock into that completely placid lake, the whole surface becomes jagged with ripples, and the pure reflection of the moon is distorted and can no longer be seen. The mirror now looks like a million pieces of broken glass.

For Yogananda, the moon symbolizes the greater force of the True Self. When it's calm on that lake, a symbol for your mind, your True Self can shine through in a clear, undistorted way. You aren't riled up by your own emotions, which can keep you from being able to see anything beyond the specific little drama right in front of you. When you start to let everything settle into calmness, you can tune in to subtle messages and intuitive ideas dropped into your mind and heart.

Have you ever had the feeling that an idea was just "given" to you? I call it a download. It happens more and more as you cultivate inner peace through your meditation practice. When you are centered, Yogananda teaches, "Calmness is the voice of God speaking to you through the radio of your soul."[5] Contrast this when life is a chaotic mess. You can't perceive much of anything, and if you can't read the signs life is giving you or the messages your body is throwing your way, you're more likely to make mistakes that can impact you, slow you down, and cause you to miss amazing opportunities or make the wrong choices. To create your best life, guess what? You have to get out of your own way and stop blocking yourself. You do this by developing calmness or inner peace.

Life-Altering Benefits of Inner Peace

- Conserve your vital energy versus deplete it and age faster
- Access more intuition-based epic ideas and solutions
- Respond instead of react (and regret it later)
- Feel centered as you move through your day
- Eliminate confusion and create clarity in your daily decisions
- Change your life more rapidly and efficiently
- Step into your true power

Imagine stillness like in the hub of a spinning car wheel. There's all of this energy spinning around the tire and radiating out when the car is in motion. But as you move from the outside of the wheel, which is churning, and you start gravitating toward the middle, you move toward a still point. In the very center of the wheel is a place of calm. The world may be moving at high speeds, but there is a very powerful point inside you, and it is from the center that the True Self can be accessed in miraculous ways.

A DIFFERENT WAY TO MAKE DECISIONS

When you live from your center, you will start to make decisions from a completely different place. Instead of focusing on outer information, which can be contradicting and confusing, you find a place of inner clarity. From this place of peace, you'll cultivate the clarity needed that will make you a decision-making expert because you will be tapping into your point of power, namely the True Self.

One of the most obvious areas in my life where I've benefited from inner peace has been with personal relationships. I must admit, I didn't have the best track record when it came to romantic relationships. I carried around a lot of doubt and confusion in my relationships, wondering if I was with the right person and then finally seeing I was not with the right person. I went into relationships sometimes reluctantly, picking someone safe and wonderful but more of a friend, or thinking I could "fix" someone into being the perfect mate. Bad idea!

Then I met Jon, my husband, during a time when I was at peace with myself. Jon was unlike anyone I had ever dated—he's kind of a cross between a teddy bear and an MMA fighter. Now, if I hadn't been at peace with myself, I might have gotten lost in outer appearances and outer activities. And we would never have gotten together. After all, Jon's body is almost completely covered in tattoos from the neck down, and I have none. He is really into lifting weights, motorcycles, mixed martial arts, and at the time we met, smoking brisket on his fancy grill—and even wearing a gold grill in his teeth! None of these are my bag. In fact, nothing about Jon could be further from the kind of guy I imagined I would end up marrying, at least based on the externals we usually focus on when we make decisions.

But I bypassed all of that on the surface. Sure, I've used outer criteria in the past to make decisions, and guess what? I made a lot of mistakes. When I met Jon at a random dinner party in Venice Beach, I was in a completely different place. Within just a few minutes of talking, I could tune right in to his energy, in to his big heart. From my heart, my center,

I found a deep, profound connection. Something that no one could see with their physical eyes, and people might even scratch their heads when they see us together, at least at first. But from the calmness of my center, my deep inner knowing told me this man was my One. This knowing— the True Self—knew what it was doing!

I'm sure you've experienced this knowing at some point in your life. Recall a time when you made a decision from a non-calm place. How did that work out for you? In contrast, recall a time when you made a decision when you were truly calm and felt centered. How did that work out differently?

Peace Now Practice

In the chaos of daily life, where are you supposed to go to get calm? Into yourself, and into your breath. You can retreat from the noisy, hectic outer world (temporarily), at any time, and center yourself within. You are powerful enough to be the sanctuary for yourself without needing anyone or anything outside of yourself. It's like scuba diving. When you jump off the boat with your gear, your inflated vest keeps you on the surface, where at first the water can be very choppy. But as you deflate your vest, you sink deeper down into the water, past the surface, and as you inch down, things start to get very still.

You may not be able to escape from work or your kids for a full meditation practice during the day, but you can take one minute to do this Peace Now Practice. If you're out in public, you can even excuse yourself to go to the restroom or to your car and do it in there! Whatever it takes. The beneficial power of inner peace on your body and mind cannot be underestimated.

Your breath is like your calmness anchor that is always with you. Yogananda teaches how the breath helps us to transcend the sensations of the body and quiet restless thoughts. Again, even in the middle of chaos. You can therefore practice this at any time—when your partner is driving you nuts, when you're worried about the bills, or after you've gotten sucked into an endless news cycle loop.

1. Find a quiet, private place (again, even if it's the bathroom, where you can close the door for 60 or 90 seconds!). Find a place where you can sit if you can, but if standing is all you can do, then go with that.

2. Close your eyes, and place one hand on your belly and one hand on your heart. Take the first moment to just check in. Notice if your heart is beating faster than normal, if your breath is only coming down into your upper chest. Whatever you find in your body, just witness it instead of judging it.

3. Now, move both of your hands to your belly. Imagine your belly is a big balloon. While counting to six, try to "inflate" your belly by breathing all the way down into your belly center. If you are really doing this, your hands should actually rise.

4. Exhale for a count of six; your belly should deflate like a balloon with the air being squeezed out of it.

5. Repeat this pattern for at least six cycles, or longer if you have time.

6. When complete, place both hands over your heart and affirm, "I am peace now." Let this sink in, and feel the energy of peace washing over you. Rest here for as long as you can, at least a few moments.

7. As always, close by bringing your hands together in prayer, or Anjali mudra, and take a moment for gratitude, giving thanks in general, or for anything specific that comes to you.

MOVING PAST NERVOUSNESS

Yogananda goes on to say that "Nervousness is the disease of civilization." And this was decades before the current anxiety epidemic of modern society! It's very depleting to overload your nerves by constantly reacting to stimuli in the outside world all day, every day, which is loud, erratic, insane, and grabbing for your attention. If you put too much attention into the ever-shifting outer world, your energy accordingly becomes ever-shifting and restless. You become like the lake with rocks tossed into it, day in and day out.

Your sympathetic nervous systems starts to go into overdrive, signaling to your adrenals to fire up, go into fight-or-flight mode, and secrete stress hormones like cortisol. Your body gets further imbalanced and inflamed, as this should not be your normal resting state. Uneasiness, confusion, and restlessness abound. These are all signs that you are definitely veering off the enlightenment path!

Instead, when you are calm, your energy can flow back into your central nervous system in your spine. Like an electrical circuit, when you turn your energy back in, it doesn't get depleted or used up. Instead, it builds in capacity. And that energy can be used to perceive new breakthrough solutions and ideas, as well as boost your vitality. We become shepherds over our own energy, carefully pointing it in the right direction. The more we stay peaceful, the less we become agitated by what's going on outside of ourselves—positive or negative—and our overactive minds start to settle down.

The center of anything is where things are most stable. It's a place of concentrated force, a place of strength. It is the place of pure potentiality where anything is possible.

Just like the sun, which beams its powerful light and heat in all directions, it is from your peaceful center that the presence and energy of the True Self radiates.

Be like the sun. Shine forth.

Practical Tips for Accessing Peace in Your Life

1. **First, make up your mind to be more peaceful.**
   It may sound basic, but intention is everything. First, you have to make a clear decision about what you want to create in your life. To find your center, as Yogananda says, "Make up your mind to be calm no matter what happens." Don't worry, the "no matter what happens" part is a work in progress for all of us, because to be honest, a lot of things can still make me feel less than calm (you know, screaming kids at 4 A.M., a virus that deletes all your e-mails . . .), but I still see progress. And what's important is committing to this intention. Right now, just decide to be calm as much as possible. You can even use the phrase "Be peace" as a mantra you can say throughout the day.

2. **Stay centered and surrendered.** Spiritually speaking, trust means that if you do your best right now in the present moment, your life will unfold as it is meant to. Buddha taught that the only way "not to be assailed by past and future" is to be mindfully present moment to moment in your life, without attachment to the outcome of your actions. Life is ever-changing, but if you can show up in the now and just be, you will

feel free no matter what happens. In this way, trust helps you to stay less attached to things having to be a certain way. So stay present, which is where your power is rooted.

3. **Take notice of how powerful you feel when you are being calm and in your center.** Sometimes we flit about our day without noticing what we are feeling. Today, pay attention to your body and how it feels during the day. Maybe traffic makes your heart race, or you notice a tightness in your shoulders before a scheduled Zoom call with your boss. Pay attention. You don't have to write anything down. Just take notice. It's like tuning in to more awareness about how certain foods make you feel after you eat them. Also, notice how your body feels when you are mentally peaceful. In this case, your goal is to become more aware of your states of being as you move through your day.

4. **Speak kindly.** Yogananda says, "Another major cause of nervousness is unkind speech. Never gossip or talk against others."[6] The more you get too entangled in the drama of daily life, the more you get distracted from focusing on your center.

   So worry less and comment less on what other people are doing. It just takes away from your power when you focus on it. It's yet another way to distort your attention and energy. Consciously avoid gossip magazines, angry news websites, and negative conversations from your life, and notice how much clearer you start to feel. Kindness is a beautiful quality that will help you feel centered.

5. **Batch your time spent on media and social media into pockets of defined times.** It could be, say, from 8–8:30 A.M., midday at 12–12:30, and at 6–7:00 P.M. It's up to you. Decide the times you are going to go in and explore. The rest of the time you stay off of it. That way, you have space to go back to your center during the day instead of continually having alerts going off that interrupt your flow to show you what's going on with everybody else's lives. It's great to connect with the community! But you can do it in a more deliberate way that allows you to know what's going on out there when you need to, and yet stay calm and centered within.

6. **Schedule less so you have more downtime.** Packing so much into each day that we're constantly running from one thing to the next is *not* conducive to calmness. It's conducive to anxiety! Ironically, you will be more productive as you slow down because you can put more of your full energy into one thing at a time, with gaps to recenter yourself.

   We've all experienced this or something similar: you are running late for a meeting, and you look all around for your car keys. You start to panic a little and start looking in the kitchen, the dining room, the bedroom. You don't find them. You panic a little more and go back and look in the same places again because maybe you missed something.

Finally, you come to a stop, take a breath, and whisper a short prayer to yourself: *Please help me find these freakin' keys, or I'm going to explode!* Something in you suggests that your keys are in your pocket. And so they are. Turns out, a touch of stillness in the midst of your little freak-out is where you found what you were looking for.

Chapter 9

YOU ARE CONFIDENCE

"You don't have to acquire anything;
you have it already. The gold of the soul is right there
within you, covered with the mud of delusion.
All you have to do is scrape off that mud."

— PARAMAHANSA YOGANANDA[1]

Confidence is a glowing quality. You can spot it from a mile away; it catches your eye. Confident people command attention. You can't help but look at them and how they walk around like a big bright light bulb. But upon closer examination, you will see that there are actually two kinds of confidence. And they are very different indeed. One kind starts to crumble pretty fast when you look at what's really behind it. And the other kind of confidence, albeit far rarer in our world, actually starts to become more glorious the closer you look, which is a sure sign of truth.

I know you probably want to feel confident in a lasting way, a way that can't easily get deflated and dinged around, the way that you may have felt in the past. Don't worry, because we are going to move past that flimsy kind of confidence and focus on the authentic kind of confidence, which is the focus of this chapter.

FALSE CONFIDENCE

Let's look at surface confidence first. The basis of this kind of confidence is rooted in materialism: money, status, material objects like houses, boats, cars, and jewelry, a beautiful face and body, even intellectual superiority. As I've mentioned earlier, material things aren't necessarily bad. Material objects do give us a certain sense of security. What I'm talking about is overconfidence in the material, or in other words attaching *all* one's confidence to the material. You might spot surface confidence in the wealthy businessman who has an ever-rotating eye-candy watch and partner-of-the-week on his arm. Or in the haughty, closed half-smile of a scantily clad woman with a killer body. Or in the smug arrogance of a hipster tech entrepreneur who made a few hundred million dollars a few years after dropping out of college. There's nothing wrong with having or being any of these shiny things, but more often than not, this type of confidence masks a deep insecurity.

Anything you can see or hold physically or quantify is by nature going to shift and change. It's limited and therefore has only a limited ability to make you feel confident. And furthermore, anything that you identify with on the surface is really a function of ego. **Yogananda teaches, "The soul is the true Self, the pure manifestation of Spirit within you. The ego is the pseudo-self, the soul responding to the world of duality while in a state of identification with the limited instruments of the physical body and mind."[2]**

When we identify with the ego, we are always going to run into limits. So that cocky businessman might feel his self-assurance tank if his investments deteriorate or the market changes. If a beautiful woman's confidence is solely derived from her appearance, she'll feel her confidence disappear over time as she ages and her looks change or if she gains a few pounds. The hipster entrepreneur loses confidence quickly if her company's tech is outdone by another's and her stock value plummets.

Even ability and intelligence, attributes of the mind, cannot be the real source of our confidence. We can *always* find people who are "above" us in external measurements—money, sales numbers, social media followers, degrees, number of published studies, job titles, you name it.

If you try to be confident from the ego, you will never feel truly confident. You will feel insecure. And insecurity leads to suffering. And really no one wants to suffer. No one.

TRUE CONFIDENCE

True confidence comes from identifying with the True Self. Period. Its power doesn't come from the outside world. Sure, we can, and may, work to improve our looks, our financial situation, or our skills. It's natural to do these things, because let's face it, we can talk as much as we want about spirituality and our souls, but we also have a physical body and there are economic and social realities that we must contend with every day. *Yet it is possible to connect to yourself far more deeply, to stop identifying with externals alone.* When we do this, real freedom begins to arise in our lives in the form of true confidence.

Embodiment, which is another word for "realization" or "integration," is an attribute of true confidence. Now, this can be a pretty abstract concept for something that is supposed to take the abstract and make it concrete! But embodiment really means you are giving form to all the great things inside you, those things that often are hidden by all the junk, baggage, old hurts, misunderstandings, and pain that you might be carrying inside of you.

This extraneous stuff often takes the form of mental chatter, which tricks you into devaluing yourself, and sometimes in a "positive way." By this I mean you might label yourself a president, a YouTube star, a tireless mother of four. And these things may be part of you, but you are more than an executive, a social media maven, or mom (as great as these personae are). You transcend all of these labels because you are the True Self. You are sacredness in action.

Of course you need to accept this birthright, which is essentially what embodiment means. Somewhere along the way, we experienced a form of amnesia and we forgot how truly special we are. Instead, we started acting like beggars or brats or wallflowers or charlatans. We have forgotten—or maybe we were just never truly taught because of circumstances or the people in our lives—that we are something truly awe-inspiring.

Embodiment means you realize that every situation counts, whether anyone is watching or not. As you become increasingly embodied, there isn't any more separation between who you are out in the world and the integrity of really being it. Living from the reality of the True Self eliminates the intense insecurity that surrounds the so-called fraud syndrome, which entails being worried that you will be "found out" for not being who you say you are. While most everyone may think that you are successful, wonderful, or whatever you project, deep down inside yourself you know that you aren't fully living it in daily life.

If you're reading this right now and saying, *Oh man, that's me.* It's okay. You're here for a reason. You're ready to go beyond just the projections. You are ready to live your truth by first deciding to be the person that you want to be and then closing the divide. You do that by making the commitment to your meditation practice and doing the self-work through the exercises in this book. You can drop all the pretense. Just start living it now.

Once the divide closes between your beliefs, truth, words, and actions, you become embodied, and you become confident in the real way. A big sign of this, which always goes along with true confidence, is exhibiting humility and kindness. All of that other crap behavior, including being snobby, snarky, and pretentious, was just the wounded ego having its day out in the sun and pretending it was confident under a veil of deep self-doubt. Being humble, on the other hand, radiates and registers as attractive and supremely powerful. As the old saying goes, the first will be last and the last will be first. Embracing humility unlocks your sacred inheritance.

When you connect to the True Self inside of you, it's the end of trying to desperately cling to fleeting surface confidence. You know that the light is working through you and coming through you in a completely unique way. The need to compare yourself to others starts to fade away like an old board game that just bores you now. When you fully connect with the real you, true confidence will take root. This brings in a stabilizing, grounding energy into your life that strengthens everything you do.

No longer will you have to question if you are good enough or peek around the room and wonder if you belong at that event or party. You belong because you are you. Yogananda urges us in this regard, "Getting along with self is the most important point in getting along in this world. So first and foremost you must learn truly to appreciate and love yourself."[3]

THE TRUTH EMERGES

No matter how much money you have or don't have in the bank, or if you aren't married yet while all your friends already have three kids, or you just have never felt truly confident, know that you can access true confidence now without having to first change anything on the outside. In fact, please, please don't focus on the outside at all at first.

Why not? Because the outside will change to align to your new energy on the inside and the resulting way you walk about the world with confidence and strength. Outer change always starts as an inside job. As you let go of chasing after false confidence, dynamic forces and energies are freed up. **Your outer world will change to match your inner world, and it's going to be so incredibly powerful for you when it starts to happen.**

When I first got home from my long backpacking trip, I would sit at the edge of my Murphy bed in my tiny apartment in New York City to study, meditate, and apply what Yogananda was teaching me. Within a short time, I began to see patterns within his teachings that led to an explosion of creativity and energy inside of me. I started placing my identity in something different, something much bigger than the small little me I had identified with until that point. My whole energy changed and radiated out a confident knowing. Manifestations began to happen. Money began showing up when I needed it. I met people who I needed to meet, which led to new opportunities. I then started writing books, which led to appearances on national television shows.

This can happen to you, too, when you identify with the light inside of you: things that seemed impossible start to come in as actualized reality. Things that felt blocked will start to open up for you. Then you will come to know as truth in your life Yogananda's wisdom: "Every human being is a representative of the Infinite Power."[4]

When Yogananda came to the United States in the 1920s, he wore traditional Indian robes and had dark brown skin. As you can imagine, he certainly encountered all sorts of prejudice from parts of the population who had never seen such a figure. He also experienced backlash from those who felt threatened about his ideas about oneness and universal truth. Yet despite any resistance he encountered outwardly, he always remained calm and secure in his message. Yogananda knew who he really was—a unique creation of spirit, just as we all are. His innate connection to Source was where his confidence originated. This is a state of conviction to which we can all aspire, a place of solid knowing, of unwavering belief in who we really are. We all have the ability to tap into this part of the True Self that provides assurance and fortitude. No one can take this confidence away or "get" it from us. It is our birthright.

You can start to shift today. And that is an important move not only for you, but for those around you. They will feel your rising confidence simply because you are more and more deeply connected to yourself, and not because of anything outside of yourself, and you can share with them about the True Self too. And that is a wonderful form of service you can offer them indeed. It is the birthright of all of us to vastly improve our entire lives by getting to really know and understand our true identity.

It is said that when Moses asked God what God's name was, the Almighty answered "Ham-Sah," or "I am that I am." A mysterious response to say the least, but one that speaks great truth.

When you start identifying with the real you, you will find that you cannot exactly put the essence of "you" into words. It's a unique energy that can only be felt and experienced from within you. In the chapter YOU ARE A CREATOR, we will explore how your unique essence gets channeled into actions and creations in the physical world, so that you can harness its fullest potential. But for now, realize that your real confidence should come from you *being* you. It's so insanely simple. Yet, as we know, simple doesn't mean easy, which is why our practice helps us do simple things in a powerful, beautiful, elegant, and profound way.

From the very quality of your presence, your Beingness emanates like a star. It's not something you have to acquire, as Yogananda so wisely teaches us in the opening quote to this chapter. It's within you. You already have the gold you're searching for. And the gold is you! You simply are! And how magnificent you truly are.

Breathing into Your True Confidence Practice

We all need reminders to connect back with our True Selves. Especially when we get triggered, which could be from anything, including your last single friend getting married, a social media post of a fancy retreat you can't afford, or your colleague getting promoted instead of you. It can be a great challenge to remember that your confidence must come from within yourself, especially in today's world, where others' journeys are constantly put right in front of your face with technology. Even though it's easy to compare yourself to others, you have to stop comparing yourself to others. Keep calling in your attention!

This can definitely be a challenge, so here's a mini breathing exercise to help you boost your confidence when you need it:

1. Find a comfortable, quiet seat. Lift and straighten your spine as you learned in Chapter 7, Practice: Meditation, Part I: Foundation.

2. Next, breathe in and silently say "I," then breathe out and silently say "Am." The mantra here is "I am." This is to affirm that you simply are you. Your confidence comes from being a unique, breathing creation in and of yourself. *Period.* End of story.

3. Continue for at least 8–10 breath cycles. Keep going until you can quiet the intrusive thoughts, and move your attention inward and feel recentered.

4. Then do a few deep breaths without the mantra. When you feel complete, close in gratitude.

YOU ARE BEYOND COMPARISON

Hishtavut is the Hebrew term for "equanimity," which means that you are unaffected by praise or scorn. Once you connect to your true confidence, you really stop caring so much what other people think of you either way. Talk about freedom!

If you know in your heart that you are acting in your truth, or as the yogic phrase says, you are taking "right action," then you know what you know, and your confidence doesn't go up and down with the outside world. **You are what you are, and no one can ever take that away from you.**

Comparing yourself to anyone else is a big no-no. First of all, it means you are identifying with your ego. It's like trying to decide what's better: an oak tree, a redwood, or a sequoia. As I write this and look out my window at those three trees in my yard, it becomes obvious that there are no comparisons in nature. No one tree is better than another.

Secondly, comparison pushes you into the dangerous world of duality. Duality is the opposite of Oneness. Duality is the feeling of "you and I are different and against each other." It's an energy that divides, so you go from feeling connected to others to making comparisons with others to contrasting differences between others and then ultimately feeling competitive with and pitted against others. Instead of leading with harmony and leaning in to your own light, your energy starts to focus more on what such and such is doing and how you can outdo them and be "better" than someone else.

It's all divisive, and you are not ultimately going to feel confident if you play that game. It just makes you feel disillusioned and separated from your sisters and brothers all around you. "You define yourself by so many different titles applicable to your body and mortal roles. . . . You must peel off these titles from the soul," teaches Yogananda.[5]

It's not to say we're naive and don't acknowledge competitive products or offerings in the world at large. Of course that exists. But if you focus on your own gifts and unique expression and the True Self, and you continue to let go of your smallness and start owning the greatness inside of you, you will find your own way to succeed. And you can do that without having to be overly concerned about what others are doing. You just focus on your path. Other people around you may still compare and identify with the outside measurements, but you are free.

When you remain centered, your foundation is solid and strong. Storms can't shake you, and disappointment is seen for what it is—a momentary setback as well as an opportunity to try something new. Confidence means knowing you have the right stuff. And having the right stuff ultimately leads to victory.

Practical Ways to Develop True Confidence in Your Life

1. **Start with small chunks of time.** For many of us, cruising on the true confidence bandwagon is going to be a bumpy ride. It's difficult to make a change, and even more difficult to make a change that involves a complete reevaluation of who we think we are and how we respond to life. So, start in increments. If you want to make a 180-degree turn, start by changing directions by just one degree. Maybe practice affirmations for a couple of minutes a day or run a positive dialogue in your head for five minutes when you wake up or go to sleep at night. Then try to increase that time every day by another minute. It might sound cliché, but slow and steady wins the race.

   You can also try this thought experiment: imagine that you bought a piano last year, and then a full year passed, and you never touched the keys. That's a year of nothing, in terms of learning to play the piano. Now imagine you practiced for ten minutes a day every day. You might not be Mozart at the end of the year, but you would have clocked in 3,650 minutes of practice. And guess what? That's over two full days (over 60 hours) of piano playing! Now imagine what your life would be like if you worked on your inner confidence for ten minutes a day for a year. What do you think would happen? My guess: you would be closer and closer to your amazing, epic dream life.

2. **Make your morning meditation the most important part of your morning routine.** As you go further along in your practice, this will not have to be a reminder. Why? Because you will start to see such an enormous difference between the days when you do and when you don't meditate! Meditation will set the tone for your whole day. It will give you the foundation of true confidence, and it will shift the way you carry yourself in the world and interact with others.

   Do not worry if you feel restless during meditation, especially when you first start out. The more you keep making the effort, the more you will be surprised at how your life begins to change. Sometimes when you are so close to something, it's hard to see little changes, like when other people comment on how much taller your kid is. You might not notice it because you see him every day, but others do.

   I remember when it hit me for the first time that my practice was changing me. It was back when I was still living in New York, and one day I just realized how different I felt. Calmer. More focused. Happier. There's no meditation benefit barometer, of course! But when I tuned in, it was undeniable—I felt better than I had in a very long time. And the same will happen for you. Then you will see your whole relationship to yourself and your confidence start to shift.

3. **Catch yourself comparing.** Anytime you start to compare yourself to another, say to yourself, *"There I go again, comparing! Not today!"* Redirect yourself back to center; take some deep breaths. Let feelings pass. No big deal! Things come up, and things can just as easily fade away. Be happy for others, remind yourself that everyone's path is unfolding in its own way, and know that your good is coming to you too.

4. **Center yourself before you go into social situations.** Try meditating and connecting to your True Self before you go into situations that are challenging for you or inspire you to slip back into comparison mode. These could be parties, industry events, conferences, or even everyday social media. Know when you are most vulnerable, and work on fortifying yourself right before. Try doing your Breathing into Your True Confidence technique, above, before any social gathering.

Chapter 10

PRACTICE:
Meditation, PART II:
THE THIRD EYE

*"The door to the kingdom of heaven is in the
subtle center of transcendent consciousness at the point
between the two eyebrows. If you focus your attention
on that seat of concentration, you will find tremendous
spiritual strength and help from within."*

— PARAMAHANSA YOGANANDA[1]

THE IMPORTANCE OF MUDRAS

Mudras refer to specific positioning of the fingers, hands, and other body parts that are used in meditation and yoga asana postures to affect your prana, your life force energy, in beneficial ways. You may have seen statues in the Eastern section of a museum or temple and wondered why the hands were placed in such specific, graceful, and beautiful ways. Now you know! Mudras are believed to be especially helpful in aiding you in redirecting your energy away from your senses to flowing inward.

One of the most powerful yogic secrets has to do with where and how you position your eyes during meditation. **Yogananda stresses that the position of your eyes during meditation is of utmost importance in increasing your access to higher wisdom and perception.** If we are going to take the time to do something—in this case, meditate—we want to be sure to do all that we can to amplify the benefits we are seeking! And these specific details matter.

Shambhavi mudra is the mudra of fixing your inner gaze toward the center and slightly up to the spot between your eyebrows, the point known as the third eye. Shambhavi is linked to Shambhu, or one of the iterations of the name Shiva, Lord of Yogis, who also represents the Supreme Self. Another name for this spot is "Shiva eye."

When we focus on this spot, it is believed to also help promote mental peace. It may feel a little unnatural or even a bit of a strain to have your eyes gaze inward in that position, but over time it will get easier and feel like second nature (of course, if you have any eye issues, avoid overly straining your eyes). Eventually, it can become like your internal happy place, where you look forward to going, and you will be able to drop into deeper and deeper stillness and calmness when you go into this mudra.

After working with this technique for a while, I feel an increasing awareness of my third eye. It's as if part of my consciousness is now being pulled up there by an internal stream of energy. And the more I connect with the third eye, the less things bother me in the world in general, because it feels like I have access to a much bigger picture. It's like being able to see through an expanded drone view versus the teeny little frame of your phone camera. You will be surprised to find as you go along in your practice, as I did, that there's a lot more to see than you ever realized.

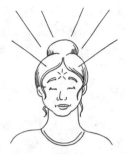

THE SIXTH CHAKRA

The word *chakra* roughly translates to "wheel" and refers to energy centers in your body. There are seven major chakras, located along your spine, that correspond to emotional, spiritual, and mental energies. They start at the base of your spine, at your root, or *Muladhara* chakra, and continue up to your crown, or *Sahasrara* chakra.

The focal point between your eyebrows is your sixth chakra, or your *Ajna* chakra. The yogis believe this to be your seat of intuition and higher knowing. And it is here that you can see far beyond what your physical eyes can see.

Yogananda teaches us that if we just believe that what we can see physically is all there is, then we remain in delusion. It's kind of like if you looked around where you are sitting right now and believed nothing existed beyond your eye line. With this mindset, we will continue to go through our lives thinking we are small, limited beings. But when we start to tune in to our third eye, we can see far, far beyond the limited material world of people and things. We can start to tune in to energy and the interconnectedness of all things, love, joy, and profound peace.

What else is there to see? For one, "seeing" can imply gleaning greater access or knowing of intuitive information and wisdom, which can be used to make the right decisions and discern the next best steps in your life. It gives you a much higher level of insight. It's practical as well as mystical. Though on that latter part, if you're open to it, the yogis also believe that it is possible, in advanced meditation, to see lights and worlds beyond this one, such as in the astral realm.

The verse Matthew 6:22 in the New Testament says, "The light of the body is in the eye: if therefore thine eye be single, thy whole body shall be full of light." Some believe that Jesus went to India during the lost years of Christ, and learned about yoga, and that this passage is an esoteric reference to the third eye.

Nonetheless, in the yogic belief system, the more you focus on your third eye, the more you can increase your higher perceptions. When you do this, you can expand your connection with the joy, power, intelligence, and love of your True Self and make these qualities more accessible to you in your day-to-day life.

Yogananda taught that real truths have to be experienced, not just read about. So let's get started with accessing your third eye.

1. **Get into the proper position in your meditation seat.** Be sure to lift and straighten your spine.

2. **Start with an intention.** Focus your mind, and dedicate your practice.

3. **Do the preliminary breathing exercise from Paramahansa Yogananda[2] of tensing and relaxing your body (described in detail in Chapter 7).** Here are some key reminders of this technique: As you inhale and hold in the breath, simultaneously tense the whole body

to a count of six. Next, expel the breath in a double exhale of "huh, huhhh," a sound made by the breath rushing out. Relax all the tension in your body at the same time. Repeat this exercise three times.

4. **Do the Expanding the Gaps Practice.** Ideally this would be at least 5–10 or more minutes, as you are getting started with your practice (more detail back in Chapter 4).

5. **Focus on your third eye.** Now, keeping your breath slow and even, while your eyes are still closed, lift your internal gaze to your third eye. This spot is between your eyebrows and slightly higher, so it will feel like a lifted gaze. Try not to strain, but to rest your gaze there with a gentle and consistent focus.

6. **Add a mantra to your third eye focus.** Keeping your inner gaze raised up to your third eye, start to repeat the simple, one-word mantra over and over again: Peace. Keep breathing, keep your internal gaze focused there, and keep repeating: Peace, Peace, Peace. You may notice that as you continue to focus on your third eye, that your breath starts to slow down and the pace at which you say the mantra does also. Let it feel like a relaxed rhythm. If your gaze drops down, just keep lifting it gently but consistently back to your third eye (stay tuned for more discussion on mantra in Chapter 18).

Continue this practice for ideally 5–10 minutes.

7. **Close in gratitude.** When you've completed your practice, bring your hands together in Anjali mudra, or prayer position, in front of your heart. As we always close our meditations, take a moment to be grateful for your breath, these teachings, and your practice, and whatever else spontaneously arises from your heart. You can also say a prayer if that resonates with you.

   Note: Ideally, your total meditation practice will grow to 20 minutes or more whenever and as often as you can. If you need to keep your practice to 10 minutes when starting out, do steps 1–5 from the foundational Chapter 7 practice, but shorten the portion dedicated to the Expanding the Gaps practice to 3 minutes or so, so you have more time to connect in with your third eye.

Chapter 11

YOU ARE AN INTUITIVE BODY

*"Intuition is soul guidance....
The goal of yoga science is to calm the mind,
that without distortion it may hear the
infallible counsel of the Inner Voice."*

— PARAMAHANSA YOGANANDA[1]

LISTENING TO YOUR HEART

As adults, we all have to make decisions, big and small, on a daily basis. And let's face it: the quality of the decisions we make determines the quality of our lives. When you make good decisions, life flows. When you make bad decisions, it doesn't. Instead of expansive, productive, and fun times, you spend a lot of energy and effort backtracking, cleaning up the mess, and trying to patch things back together.

We all make mistakes, of course. And we all have blind spots, the areas of life where we seem to consistently make bad decisions. One of my big fat blind spots has been around picking romantic partners, as I've already shared with you. Luckily none of the guys I've been in relationships with have been jerks. They actually are wonderful people. But that doesn't mean we were compatible.

I'm someone who needs and values closeness. I like to snuggle right in there, physically and emotionally, and be totally open with my partner about my feelings, dreams, fears, the whole lot. But in the past, I've picked some partners who weren't on that same wavelength. Sure, there was attraction, and we would get along well in many ways; we knew some of the same people, worked well socially, and even shared the same interests, such as traveling to experience interesting cultures and being outdoors.

Yet, with some of these partners, there always seemed to be an emotional wall that separated us. We could experience a certain level of intimacy, but I never felt completely comfortable being myself. This created a pattern in my life: fall in love, have good times, but never reach that depth that I wanted. Later, after a breakup, I would scratch my head and think, "Hmm, wonder why I thought he was a good choice?" Of course, I really didn't have to ponder too deeply, because even though my head was confused, my heart was always telling me, *He's not the one.*

When it comes to love, we don't always have clear vision, because our brains often talk over our hearts. And the heart is the seat of intuition; it's the foundation for our emotional intelligence. Let me stress the word *intelligence*, because the heart is smart (I'm going to make that into a bumper sticker). It often knows better than our brains, which tend to act like a wild frat boy with a couple of six packs and a box of condoms driving his father's convertible at high speeds, goading you on: *Screw it. Have fun. Keep going. Don't listen to the heart! Party on, y'all!*

Still, the heart in all its intelligence stays calm and tries to communicate with us. Intuition does this in subtle ways. We might get a feeling inside—it's kind of like a tiny push that we feel in our chest or back that is trying to get our attention. It might be a quiet voice that tries to call out to us in the midst of brain chatter. But if we don't know that's our intuition talking to us, we can ignore these sensations and let the brain take us for a ride.

You might have fun for a little while, but along the way you pick up a scorching case of herpes, lose all your money, and now have a criminal record in Tijuana. Maybe it's time to rethink—refeel—things, and the next time your brain is stopped at a red light, thrust the car into park, grab the keys, and kick the putz (your brain) to the curb. Heart's driving tonight, bitch!

You can develop your intuition now. Even after you make, well, a few detours. "Mistakes" are an important part of our journey because they further motivate us to get back to center, whether we consciously realize that or not. We don't want to keep feeling the same pain from the same patterns, so we put more energy into doing things differently.

Back in the Fearlessness chapter, I described my reset period where I hunkered down for five months to reset (and just so you know, I was still working and taking care of my family, but I was also reallocating my time to refill what I had emptied out for a few years). I was meditating and studying and doing my practice, which it turns out, is the key to developing your intuition. Yogananda says, "The surest way to liberate the expression of intuition is by meditation, early in the morning and before going to bed at night."[2]

Some months after being in my self-imposed quasi-isolation period, I found myself at that random dinner party of about 12 people. And one of them turned out to be Jon, my future hubby. As you read before, Jon, at first blush, wasn't necessarily my type, but I had learned to silence frat-boy brain so much that my heart, my intuition was saying, *He's the one! He's the one!*

I've found that intuition is one of the most important things we can develop in our lives, because it relates to all our decisions that make up the fabric of our day-to-day experience.

Self-Reflection: Tuning in Your Way

How does your intuition communicate with you, exactly? Is it a thought in your mind? A feeling in your body? If so, where in your body does that feeling occur? And what exactly does it feel like?

FEELING INTO INTUITION

Intuition really isn't that difficult to understand. We might call it a hunch, but we're not aware of the thousands if not millions of bits of information that we are experiencing at any moment and that are being processed by the brain and our nervous system. Our bodies are intuitive powerhouses.

Think about how inflammation works: we cut ourselves, and white blood cells take off to fend off intruders, whether it's a paper cut or a gunshot wound. We don't tell them to do anything; they just do it. And our bodies and minds are constantly doing these things to protect us, things that we call intuition. From a spiritual perspective, meditation helps us to differentiate our all-knowing True Self and our own judgments, prejudices, and habits that often override our underlying awareness or True Self.

Intuition—the idea that individuals can make successful decisions without deliberate analytical thought—has intrigued philosophers and scientists alike since the times of the ancient Greeks. There is more and more research emerging about the viability and importance of intuition in the scientific community.

Case in point: researchers from the University of New South Wales have now studied intuition and demonstrated just how much unconscious intuition can inform—and even improve—our decision-making. "These data findings suggest that we can use unconscious information in our body or brain to help guide us through life, to enable better decisions, faster decisions, and be more confident in the decisions we make," researcher Joel Pearson says.[3]

Gerd Gigerenzer of the Max Planck Institute for Human Development in Berlin says that people rarely make decisions on the basis of reason alone, especially when the problems faced are complex. He believes intuition's merit has been vastly underappreciated and views intuition as a form of unconscious intelligence.[4] In their 2006 paper, Ap Dijksterhuis and his colleagues, then at the University of Amsterdam, also concluded that intuition was valuable. The researchers tested what they called the "deliberation without attention" hypothesis: although conscious thought makes the most sense for simple decisions, it can actually be detrimental when considering more complex matters, such as buying a house.[5]

As *Psychology Today* points out, scientists use creative intuition to select which paths to follow toward potential discoveries. Nobel laureates have discussed their use of hunches. Michael S. Brown, an American geneticist who was awarded the Nobel Prize in Physiology or Medicine, has said, "As we did our work, I think, we almost felt at times that there was almost a hand guiding us."[6]

Self-Reflection:
Your Personal Relationship to Intuition

Spend a few minutes journaling the answers to these questions:

1. Do you have a history of tuning in to your intuition or disregarding it and your "inklings"?

2. Is there an instance you can recall when you listened to your intuition and took a different (and ultimately wonderful) path or made a beneficial decision?

3. Have you ever bypassed your brain and listened to your heart? What happened?

4. Is there an instance when you ignored your intuition and made a mistake or went down a pathway that wasn't right for you?

5. Do you know anyone you would describe as intuitive? What makes them seem so to you?

HOW DO WE DEVELOP OUR INTUITION?

Yogananda does not ever tell us to accept things blindly. He says that "constructive doubt in regard to Divine matters will move us toward truth more quickly than will dogmatic belief."[7] He urges us to test the definite meditation methods for ourselves, which have been demonstrated and replicated by yogis for centuries, to move from merely discussing beliefs to *knowing* truth by direct experience. Dogmatic belief doesn't give us clarity, and eventually, if something is off, we rebel and reject those ideas.

It's kind of like a tiny splinter you might get embedded in your hand. It might be too small to see, but you feel its irritation. You know something is wrong. Amazingly, over time your body will literally push that splinter, that thing that doesn't belong in you, out of your body. Of course, this can take time, yet it's part of your body's natural ability to take care and protect itself.

The same holds true for our emotions. If something isn't right inside you emotionally, your heart will try to get rid of it. You will feel something, but you need to pay attention and use that message to help yourself as best as you can. **Meditation heightens our awareness, which helps us to make better decisions.** And sometimes, we can't do everything on our own. Meditation allows us to know when to reach out for help. That might mean talking to a friend or a professional and discerning the best course of action.

When I initially started this path, I had the same questions that most of us have. *How do I know all of this yogic stuff is right? How do I know meditation is going to work?* How do I know this is the best path to follow for my meditations? Test it for yourself. When I found this path, I did as Yogananda told me to do: namely, question everything. I tested the ideas within myself, and I tested the meditation practice to see what arose from my own intuition and knowing. I also tuned in to see if anything was evolving or shifting within me.

And things were on the move. I was making progress and feeling shifts inside of me. I didn't follow blindly. My intuition was also developing in general across my life, and I was going beyond simply relying on hard facts to leaning on my gut instincts. For example, when I had to make the decision to move from New York to Los Angeles, at first I was worried about leaving my friends and family and life on the East Coast. Yet I listened to my inner voice, made the move, and my whole life started opening up from then on.

GO BEYOND YOUR LIKES AND DISLIKES

Something that will also help you be open to more intuition is to not become so rigid about exactly how you want everything to go. Yogananda says, "Perfect control of feeling makes you king of yourself. . . . Start by not catering to likes and dislikes."[8] The issue with being so attached to our likes and dislikes is that we become restless, which Yogananda calls a kind of "persistent discontent stirred by feeling."[9] It means that everyday things, as small as preferring a particular table at a restaurant or wanting the dishes to be put away in a certain way, can have the power to ruin your day. If we get overinvolved in the everyday minutiae, we lose sight of the big picture.

When we focus on all our little preferences, what we are really doing is reinforcing the ego, or the little self. The smaller part of us that wants things a very specific way spends enormous energy defending one's opinions and positions. The True Self, the *big* part of you that is just bursting to come out, is so much more than the daily little humdrum things. The True Self is focused on the big picture, the inner Bliss, or pure happiness.

When you tune in to the True Self, it's impossible to be overly concerned with outside circumstances and events. This doesn't mean that you can't get excited over a new pair of shoes, redecorating a room in your house, or going out to dinner with a friend, but when you connect to your inner Bliss first, you'll find that much of what seemed so important is actually pretty small. It also means that a casual movie night with your significant other can explode into one of the most memorable and joyful times in your life. Inner Bliss elevates exterior experience to new and incredible levels.

So what exactly does this mean in the real world? It means that it's okay to have preferences for how you want things to be, yet at the same time be open to what is flowing your way. When you stay open, you can make friends with the present moment, and then you can take the right action going forward, including if you want to change things. But it's key to remain open. And to not close up like a clam if something isn't exactly the way you want it. If you're only looking for hot blonde surfer types, what if your soul mate happens to be a dark-haired guy in a suit, and you walk right by him? What if your best product idea is from the suggestion that you ignored because it came from your intern instead of from your manager?

To be open is a true quality of enlightenment. Being open means we surrender to the truth that we simply don't know everything. It means we let Spirit speak to us through our intuition instead of just pushing our agenda. It means we humble ourselves to the True Self, the great force helping to guide us, direct us, and show us *the* way. Openness means we are ready and willing to experience the fullest, best expression of wherever we happen to be. We work with life's flow instead of fighting against it.

Self-Reflection: Observing vs. Judging

Constant judgment is exhausting. The more we let things just be, the more we quiet ourselves down so that our intuition can really speak to us and discern truth and the next best steps to take. As Yogananda teaches us, *"The only way to know and to live in truth is to develop the power of intuition."*[10]

Whenever you catch yourself making a judgment, like, "He needs to go on a diet!" or "Whoa! Did she use a whole bottle of hair spray today?" try to just observe and be the witness, staying as neutral as possible. We are still going to judge to a certain extent, because that's human nature. And sometimes we do of course have to make decisions that rely on our preferences. Yet in most cases, we can chill with all the judgment. Here are some examples of mental shifts you can start to make:

<u>Judgment</u>	<u>Observation</u>
That red hat she's wearing is hideous.	There's a lady wearing a red hat.
It's so much better to lift weights than to run.	Some people like to lift weights, some like to run.
There's Ruby! Looks like she gained a couple of pounds.	There's Ruby!
Ugh, it's gross and terrible when it's this hot. Just awful!	It's hot today.
That guy must be rich— he's driving a Bentley.	There's a guy in a Bentley.
She's so desperate for attention in her social media posts.	There's a social media post.

When you start to do this practice, you may be startled by how many judgments you make in a day and then a week, a month, a year! So many of those are unnecessary and can pull us off center when we're constantly making little evaluations and comparisons of the ego. Instead, keep working toward simply witnessing, and notice how much easier it becomes to listen to your intuition.

INTUITION IS THE PRECURSOR TO FAITH

The Sanskrit word for "faith" is *visvas*. It translates to "breathe easy, have trust, and be free from fear." But Yogananda says this is not the full meaning. "Svas" refers to the motions of breath, implying life and feeling, while "vi" means "opposite" or "without."[11] So it would seem that when we are calm, we can access our intuition. And developed intuition gives rise to faith because we know intuition will have our back. For those who are emotionally restless, though, accessing intuition and comprehension of the truth can be difficult or perhaps impossible. It's like the surface of that jagged lake we talked about earlier. In that state, it's impossible to see the moon's reflection. That is, until the restlessness gives rise to calmness. Equanimity proceeds intuition, which we focused on back in Chapter 8, YOU ARE PEACE.

When it is developed sufficiently, intuition brings comprehension of truth. Yogananda teaches us, "In the calmness of meditation your consciousness will be able to focus on truth and understand. In that state faith develops; through unfolding intuition you receive 'the evidence of things not seen.'"[12] Over time, as we continue to meditate and follow our practice, clarity emerges.

Practical Ways to Increase Your Intuition in Your Life

1. **Ask Spirit to guide you.** My favorite prayer for guidance is an adaptation of one that Yogananda teaches: *Spirit, I will reason, will, and act, but guide my reason, will, and actions to the highest and best things you want me to do.* This helps me set my intention of staying open to access my highest intuition, with no preconceived notions.

2. **Before making any decisions, tune in.** By tuning in, I mean to at least temporarily ignore outer voices and external influences before you make decisions. Go inside. Meditate and then listen to messages in the way of a "gut feeling" or knowing. "But if you are guided by attunement with God, He will help you do the right thing, and to avoid mistakes," teaches Yogananda.[13]

3. **Go with the flow.** In everyday life, try not to get so caught up in chasing your likes and dislikes, so that your intuition can actually guide you. Getting locked into your preferences can close off possibilities. If the restaurant is out of your dish, just get another one. If the color you wanted for your yoga pants is out, go with the good ole grey ones. Stuck at a traffic light? Use that time to meditate for a few moments. It is so liberating to free yourself of daily annoyances tied to your preferences!

4. **Notice rigidity and drop it.** Look with your flashlight of self-awareness at ways in your everyday life where you can open up more. Remember that the more open you are without strict, preconceived notions, the more you can hear your intuition speaking. Maybe you have very set ideas about specific topics or ways of going about doing something. I remember that I used to get annoyed if someone on my team didn't send over a document formatted in the "right" way. But her way wasn't wrong; it was just a different way from mine. When I let the rigidity go of wanting things to be just so, I actually started enjoying the other way. Try it! It's so freeing, and it can even be fun.

5. **Realize you can access deeper knowing.** Fully realize that you aren't an insignificant little being and don't have to make decisions from a constricted, narrow place. From the connection of the True Self, you are connected to all, including to all wisdom and a vast knowing. Tune in to that and know that as Yogananda says, "Every time you look at your body of flesh and bones, you see yourself as small and limited. If even a little thing happens to your body—if you start sneezing, or if you hit your hand hard and break it you realize your smallness. But when you close your eyes in meditation, you see the vastness of your consciousness—you see that you are in the center of eternity."[14]

Chapter 12

YOU ARE A POWERHOUSE

"The secret of vitality, therefore,
is to conserve the energy you have and to bring
new energy into the body by will power."

— PARAMAHANSA YOGANANDA[1]

Did you know that a human body at rest produces about 100 watts of power?[2] That's the equivalent of a pretty powerful light bulb that could illuminate an entire room.

And yet many of us don't feel radiant, and instead sometimes feel like we have no energy at all. There are many reasons for this—lack of sleep, improper diet, anxiety, or disease. Yet none of these states of being or conditions negates the fact that you are a power-generating body. Who you are is pure energy, pure vitality!

In this chapter, we will learn how to access and direct the vital power within you. And we're going to discuss how you can bring in more energy so that you can be a super power station who is able to create a beautiful and fulfilling life. First, a little background.

WHAT EXACTLY IS VITALITY?

Vitality is derived from the word *vita*, which means "life." From a yogic standpoint, vitality is when the life force, or prana, flows through you in abundant quantities. You feel focused, resilient, strong, confident, inspired, and unstoppable. Your skin glows, you have a bounce in your step, you laugh more, and you connect better with others. Vitality fuels your ability to be a powerhouse. The two are intimately connected.

The first person who comes to mind when I think of vitality is my Ayurvedic teacher, Vaidya Jay. When I was interning at the Ayurvedic clinic, he would show up every week not just smiling, but also humming mantras all day. Humming! Even with numerous responsibilities, a packed schedule, and a two-hour commute (or more) to Beverly Hills, he was always in a good mood. This is not hyperbole. I don't think I have ever seen him stressed. Even though he was in his late 40s, his black hair had not one spot of gray (and no, he doesn't use Just for Men), and his eyes twinkled as he bounced around to different treatment rooms. He loves vita. In other words, he loves life. He embodies vitality and is the definition of a powerhouse.

Here's the kicker, though: Vaidya Jay sleeps only about four hours every night. He is up well before sunrise every morning to do his full yoga and meditation practice, and then he hits the road. He would often tell me that he gets most of his energy from his meditations, and that, regretfully, most people don't know how to incorporate a daily mindfulness or stillness practice into their lives. If folks did, he would say, if they just learned to use their will and spend some time concentrating on how to put it to good use, it would literally change their entire world.

TURNING THE WILL INWARD

Vaidya Jay brings up a very good point. Namely, the power of our will.

Our will is basically the ability to decide to do something in our minds and then taking the steps to create it. More often than not, when we talk about will we are talking about willpower, the ability to get something done, for instance, knitting a sweater or starting a new business. And even more often, we talk about willpower as something negative, usually as a deficiency within us. "Oh, I didn't have enough willpower to stay on a healthy diet . . . I didn't have the willpower to keep up with my workouts."

But Yogananda taught that the will is something that can boost our vitality. Will is the bridge that links our individual life force energy and the greater energy of everything else. He demonstrated that there is a connection between will and energy, and that *will expands energy.*

In other words, we can use our will to access and create vitality inside of us and radiate that glowing energy out into the world. We can learn to use our will to channel more energy into our bodies through our practice and yogic techniques. In fact, yogic practices have now been studied formally and have been found, among other physical benefits, to help positively regulate systolic and diastolic blood pressure,[3] while other research has found a correlation with blood pressure and fatigue.[4] From this we can infer that healthy, regulated blood pressure will create the opposite of fatigue—vitality!

What does this mean? That our meditation practices can help us to regulate our vitality. They make us efficient. So instead of wasting our energy—like when we are home alone and have every light on in all our rooms—we can conserve our vitality to create the lives we all want.

Food, Yogananda teaches, is one source from which human beings derive energy for the body. Oxygen, sleep, and sunlight are others. But beyond these, Yogananda teaches that a main source of energy, which we can pull from at any time, is actually obtained through a point at the base of our brains called the medulla oblongata. We already touched on this way back in our first practice chapter, Chapter 4, but to review: the medulla oblongata region of your brain connects to your spine, which connects to other parts of your nervous system, including the peripheral nervous system.[5] This is said to be the exact point where energy is pulled into our bodies through the definite meditation techniques of ancient Kriya Yoga.

This energy that comes into us through meditation is always around us and omnipresent throughout the entire universe. In fact, science has proven that seemingly solid matter is actually 99.9999999+ percent space. Imagine a vast empty room with a single apple in the middle. Yet all this space isn't actually "dead space." It's not actually empty; it's pulsating with kinetic and potential energy!

Yogananda has a chant entitled, "I am the Bubble, Make Me the Sea." It illustrates this whole idea perfectly. We may think we are isolated beings cut off from everything else by our skin, which is the flimsy bubble-like boundary between us and the rest of the world, and seemingly us and the Infinite. But you literally are so much more. You are the sea of vast energy. It's something Deepak Chopra likes to call an ocean of pure potentiality. The energy that permeates you is everywhere. You really aren't cut off from the world! You and I are in it and part of it and comingled with it! We just need to learn how to direct the energy that runs through us.

Think of it this way: imagine jumping into a beautiful ocean and swimming beneath the surface. You have literally become one with the ocean. Your body is surrounded by water. Your movement affects the movement of the fish in this water, and as any skilled swimmer or surfer knows, you can harness the energy of the waves to move from place to place. We can do this aboveground too, by directing our prana, our life force.

Ayurvedic medicine, the sister science to yoga, outlines this with its *Panchamahabhuta* theory, which states that the five elements in our body: earth (*prithivi*), water (*jala*), fire (*agni* or *tej*), air (*vayu*), and ether or space (*akasha*) are the same elements found in nature. The energy of you is part of the whole, and vice versa.

We may not really pay attention to this supply of energy or realize that we *can* actually draw more of it into our bodies with our will, but that is one of the fundamental Kriya Yoga teachings. This intelligent energy is the basis of all matter. Energy is used to create all things, including building the life force vitality in your body.

I realize that I might be sounding a little too esoteric right now (but I love this stuff!), so let's do a preliminary exercise right now to demonstrate the connection between will and energy.

Connecting Intention, Will, and Energy Practice

Energy flows where we put our attention and intention. This practice will start to tie together your intention, will, and energy. Intention is a conscious aim that you create. This could be as basic as deciding to brush your teeth or clean out a closet. Or your intention could be to transform your life so you can travel the world. Intention, however, isn't a happy wish. It is a commitment to do or be something.

Your intention can direct your will, or your strength and ability to actually carry out the steps to create your intention. Your will, depending on its level of strength (which you can build through directed practice and focus), can then direct energy to create more flow in the spiritual, mental, and physical pathways in the body. This will allow the release of bound-up energy, which can otherwise cause stagnation in our minds and bodies. Here's what to do.

1. Close your eyes for a moment and set the intention for the purpose of releasing tension from your body and your mind.

2. As you inhale through your nose, imagine you are gathering all the tension that exists in your life and directing it to your shoulders.

3. For a count of three, start to increase the tension in your shoulders as you start to lift them up toward your ears. Pause at the top for a moment, and then with a big exhale out through your mouth, drop your shoulders down, and with the breath, feel the release of all the tension out of your shoulders and out of your body.

4. Repeat this three times. When you're finished, resume your normal breathing and sit quietly for a moment at least before getting up.

So, what did this demonstrate? That you have the ability to move energy in your body. And if you have the ability to move energy in your body, then you have the ability to release the feelings and sensations that don't serve you in your life and that you don't want to continue to carry.

WHAT DEPLETES VITALITY

Let's talk about a few big ways that our vitality can become depleted, which then prevents you from being the powerhouse you were born to be. Depleted vitality means you don't have as much life force to play with your kids, get through your inbox of e-mails, or walk your dog. It also means your body wears down and decomposes on a cellular level more quickly, which can lead to accelerated aging and even disease.

Everything is energy, and less energy means less life force overall; it means less rejuvenation; it means less renewal. You're like a car tire with a tiny hole in it. You can keep filling it up with air, but the tire won't stop deflating until you plug that hole.

One big vitality leak Yogananda and other yogis cautioned against happens through unrestrained emotions. When we become angry, intensely fearful, or overly anxious, we end up dispelling a ton of energy and we end up feeling drained and depleted.

Have you ever felt absolutely exhausted after an argument? It's no wonder. Research finds that emotional exhaustion is linked to a decline in attention, memory, and executive function, which involves planning and organizing.[6] Emotional upset can manifest in us physically, including aggravated digestive issues, headaches, weight loss or gain, and so on. It doesn't mean that we aren't supposed to feel our feelings.

On the contrary, we want to feel our feelings and let them pass through us, similarly to how we digest our food. Then we can emerge more calmly and address anything that needs to be addressed with poise and reason. Not only do we hear our True Selves more clearly when we are calm and in control of ourselves, but we don't wear ourselves out with unnecessary emotional extremes.

THE IMPORTANCE OF FEELING YOUR FEELINGS

Our feelings and emotions can often feel like they are controlling our lives; they can feel so wild and unpredictable and strong. When we learn to become free of them, through a process I like to think of as "digesting emotions," we can experience an enormous increase in energy in our lives and more freedom, or the very enlightenment we are seeking.

In modern society, starting from a very young age, we are not often taught to really feel our feelings. Instead, we are taught that we need to quell them, distract ourselves away from them, or push them down and ignore them. We are taught that some feelings are "negative," and so we should pretend we never have them, or at least not acknowledge them.

The issue with this is that we don't really process them, and unresolved feelings often stay in our bodies and in our lives. According to psychologist Dr. David Hawkins, author of *Letting Go,* the three major ways most people handle their negative feelings (fear, anger, sadness, jealousy, and so on) is either to suppress them, project them onto others, or avoid them through escape.[7]

When we suppress our feelings and push them down, they don't go away. Instead, they build up and create a pressure that can be felt as tension across our body (especially in the neck and back), irritability and moodiness, insomnia, digestive issues, and many other physical manifestations, like acne, pains in our joints, and headaches.[8]

Projecting our unprocessed emotions can have a destructive effect on ourselves and our relationships. This is something I know about firsthand. Today, the journey continues for me, but I have learned not to attach myself to my emotions as much. Don't get me wrong. Sometimes I slip and find myself falling back into old patterns. For instance, I remember talking to a client about the importance of self-love when a text came through on her phone. Her eyes shifted from me to the phone, and she picked up her phone and quickly texted someone back. This irritated me so much I could feel steam coming out of my ears à la a *Tom and Jerry* cartoon.

Unless it's a dire emergency, which it wasn't, two people who are having a conversation should honor and focus on each other, not on their incoming text messages. But I've learned to quickly catch myself and redirect my energy in a more positive way when a trigger goes off. I might make a joke or just let it slide. That day I just took a breath and internally wished her peace. Instead of seeing a trigger as truth, I simply notice that uneasy feelings are coming from an old wound. I breathe through the minor disturbance instead of getting caught up in it.

Finally, we all know what escape looks like. It's the face of avoidance and distraction in all its forms: alcohol, zoning out in front of the TV for hours, shopping, talking, going on social media, and so on. It's not that any of these things are wrong or bad—it's about how we use them and how much of a role they play in our lives.

PROCESSING YOUR FEELINGS

Processing feelings to digest them within ourselves means that we can feel them fully and communicate them outwardly in a neutral and not overcharged, emotional way. This allows us to conserve our energy and create a place of peace within us so we can direct it in more positive ways. Creating a personal environment of stillness is healthy and so important on our path to enlightenment.

To do that, as Hawkins explains, all we have to do is stay with a feeling until it runs its full course.[9] This is easier said than done, of course, but what Hawkins suggests is that we don't resist an emotion from rising inside of us. This act of suppression actually forces us to contain something that's not good for us. It's like having too much salt in our bodies, which can lead to water retention. It's good to have water in us, but when we retain more water than we need, it can lead to a whole list of physical ailments from bloating to contributing to high blood pressure.

So instead of retaining or blocking a feeling, bypass the rationalizations of the mind as it tries to defend your stance for feeling slighted or betrayed. Just feel, and feel, until the energy of our feelings naturally dissipates, which usually takes only a few minutes. How do you know the difference between thoughts and feelings? Feelings are wordless. They are just sensations, and you don't have to label them, as in, "Yikes, there's anger again!" Thoughts are constructs and ideas. So to process feelings, let the sensations come and go, and feel increasingly free from them. This allows inner freedom, or enlightenment, to grow more in our lives.

Self-Reflection: Your Held Emotions

Take a few minutes to write the answers to these questions in a journal. You can simply reflect on them, but writing out your responses helps you to better clarify your experiences. This is just a polite way of saying, write them down!

1. What are some negative emotions that seem to come up again and again for you?

2. What are some of your triggers? By this, I mean what are some situations that seem to come up that repeatedly bring up negative emotions in your daily life? It could be as simple as when your friends don't text you back right away or when your co-worker talks to you in what you perceive to be a bossy tone or so on. Feel into this.

3. Close your eyes and place your hands on your belly for a few moments. Ask the center of your body, "What emotions am I holding on to and not releasing?" See if your body has any wisdom to share with you at this time. It might feel weird to ask your body, and maybe you don't really get anything. That's okay. Just the practice of turning inward is important to creating deep self-connection, which is where you will find your full radiance start to grow.

OTHER VITALITY LEAKS

We also deplete our vitality through using all our time and energy in what Yogananda calls "useless activities." "Useless" might seem like a harsh word, but Yogananda was referring to pastimes that don't serve a purpose in carrying us toward enlightenment, such as excessive web-surfing, TV binge-watching, and gossip. It's okay to have down time and have fun. Actually, for all of us not-completely-enlightened beings, it is a must! Maybe when we are fully enlightened, we will have no need at all for any entertainment. But for the rest of us on the path, we definitely need a break from time to time.

The key, though, is to make sure you put aside enough time for your practice and meditations, and to keep what Yogananda deemed these other activities in check. Let's say if the only thing you ever do in the evenings after work is watch TV or movies, you would be squandering a lot of your energy on screen time. So, if you like TV, then of course you can watch it, but limit how much time you spend in front of the tube. Be sure to turn it off so you have enough time to do your meditation and practices and to spend reading or hanging out with your friends and family. The same rule applies to texting, social media time, and online shopping. Be discerning so that you can do such activities but also focus on your inward practices.

Another way we drain vitality can be through physical blockage. Yogananda taught to avoid constipation at all costs, because the accumulated toxic buildup depletes our vitality.

Yogananda also recommends avoiding eating meat (or at least overeating it), as it "loads the body with poisons" and is ultimately depleting. This is one of the reasons that pretty much all yoga masters across the board teach about following a vegetarian diet. When I learned about the energetic principles of yoga, I made the decision to become plant based.

And finally, talking too much depletes your life force. Unless you have something you really want to say, it's better to rest your voice and your energy.

VITALITY CAN GROW AT ANY POINT IN YOUR LIFE

Is it any wonder most people you see seem to have less and less radiance over time instead of having more? Without a path and tools to fuel us to be the powerhouse we were designed to be, most people live lifestyles centered around their work, organizing the many aspects of running a family or household, engaging in activities to relax that may actually deplete their vitality, and not having a practice to work with their energy in a rejuvenating way. But it doesn't have to be that way! And your vitality is not dependent on your age. As you learn to harness more energy, you can start to *grow* in vitality over time.

I've seen this to be true for my best friend and business partner, John Pisani, who now follows Yogananda's yogic teachings. When he started out, he was often stressed, tired, and run down. But now, years later, his eyes are shining, and he walks with a bounce and with grace. Everything about him feels lighter. His hair and skin look healthier, and he has more natural energy.

When you start learning to use your will more and more to draw in more energy, you will find that you may need less energy from outside sources, especially from food. I have definitely found this to be true in my own life. The more I meditate, the less dependent on food I feel. I used to have some pretty big food cravings, and like most of us, have relied on foods in the past at times to help me feel better and shift my mood.

As I go along this path, I realize I am in much better control of my moods, and I have so much energy from meditation that I don't reach for foods to boost my moods or my energy the way I used to. I'm not talking about eating food when I'm actually hungry. I'm talking about eating when I'm trying to somehow make myself feel better. Instead, now I often do mini meditations throughout the day when I need a boost. They take me a lot further than the temporary sugar highs of the past!

Improving the access to your own true vitality might not happen right away. Practice means that it continues to develop and unfold over time. But eventually you might find as you go deeper in your meditations that as Yogananda says, "The magic method of working without fatigue lies in the use of your will power."[10] The exercise in the next chapter will teach you just how to draw energy from the field that is all around us and interconnects all of us.

Summary: Supporting Your Inner Powerhouse

Boosts Vitality & Prana	**Depletes Vitality & Prana**
Meditation	Unrestrained emotions
Calmness and stillness	Too much idle time
"Digesting" your feelings	Worrying or holding grudges
Using your will for worthy pursuits	Overtalking

Chapter 13

PRACTICE:
How to Supercharge
Your Vitality

*"For will is the great suction pump of energy,
which irresistibly draws the cosmic life energy into the
body to renew it. The greater the will, the more
limitless is the supply of energy in the body."*

— PARAMAHANSA YOGANANDA[1]

First, let's call out something important upfront: the more energy that flows through your body in its deepest capacity, the more energy will flow through your life. This powerful energy is the force to fuel your creations and help transform your life.

Kriya Yoga deals directly with energy and consciousness, and focuses on pranayama, control of the life force, and meditation rather than the physical postures, such as Virabhadrasana (warrior pose) or Vrikshasana (tree pose), or other poses that you usually think of when you hear the word *yoga*.

However, as part of the Kriya Yoga science that Yogananda teaches, there is a "physical" part of the practice that involves consciously using your will to tense and relax different body parts, which Yogananda explained helps to direct energy to the body parts and increases the rejuvenation and vitality in that area of your body. We've used the practice of tensing and relaxing in some of our prior preliminary practices, but in this chapter, we go into further detail about it.

The aim of this practice is not to build muscles or flexibility, but to learn to direct and amplify the prana life force internally with the use of your will and recharge your cells, which is similar, Yogananda teaches, to recharging a car's battery with a generator.

First, it's important to understand how your energy works in the first place. There are five ways in which prana life force energy moves throughout your body, known as *prana vayus. Vayu* means "direction of energy." [2]

Prana: Governs intake, including the force of drawing the breath inward (inhaling), inspiration, forward momentum

Apana: Governs elimination, downward and outward movement, including the exhaling part of the breath

Samana: Governs absorption, assimilation, distribution of nutrients, discernment, consolidation

Udana: Governs growth and formation, speech, expression, and upward movement

Vyana: Governs circulation on all levels, as well as pervasiveness and expansiveness

What follows is a basic technique involving your will that will help you draw more energy inward and support your health and vitality. Yogananda provides deeper instruction for how to move prana throughout the body in his Energization Exercises, which are detailed in the *Self-Realization Fellowship Lessons* (see Resources for more information).

This practice involves consciously generating tension. Tension is the result of using the will to transmit energy into the muscles of your body. The greater the amount of tension you exert, the greater the energy you are calling in to your body, and into specific areas of your body.

Expanding Vitality Practice

1. Sit quietly in your meditation seat, either cross-legged on a cushion or blanket beneath your hips, or on a chair with your feet flat on the ground.

2. Begin by lifting and straightening your spine, and relaxing your breath into long, deep inhales and exhales.

3. State your intention to yourself—namely to recharge and revitalize the body. You can offer that up to the personalized form of greater intelligence/the universe/love that you connect with, if that resonates with you.

4. Practice this basic technique from Yogananda:[3]

    First, throw out the breath with a strong double exhalation (one short and one long breath). Then, inhale in a double inhalation (one short and one long breath), filling the lungs as full as is comfortable. Hold the air in the lungs for a few seconds, allowing the oxygen to be fully absorbed and converted into prana. Then repeat the double exhalation, followed by the double inhalation.

Practice this method in the fresh air 30 times in the morning and 30 times at night. It is very simple. You will be healthier than ever if you follow this. This exercise brings in a great deal of extra life force, and also decarbonizes your blood, promoting calmness.

5. When you are done, keep resting in your seat for a few moments at least, taking some deep breaths. This is now an ideal time to do the rest of your meditation practice, outlined in Chapter 10: Practice: Meditation, Part II: The Third Eye.

Chapter 14

YOU ARE BEAUTY

"We must cultivate wisdom, and learn through our wisdom to love the beauty of God in all souls and in all things."

— PARAMAHANSA YOGANANDA[1]

THE DIVISIVE PERSPECTIVE OF BEAUTY

Four of my other books have the word *beauty* in the title. It's an important topic for me, and my perspective of beauty has evolved over the years. Especially when I started to really focus on bringing Yogananda's teachings into everything I do.

There is one Yogananda quote in particular that has stayed with me for a long time: "The soul is absolutely perfect, but when identified with the body as ego, its expression becomes distorted by human imperfections."[2] Preach it, Yogananda! He's so right. If we fixate on our surface appearance, we are going to find imperfections in spades! Look at my dry skin! Where did that pimple come from? Is that a gray hair?! It's beyond frustrating!

I've experienced that extreme frustration firsthand. For years, I did not feel beautiful. I felt the complete opposite: ugly and strange-looking (growing up, I was pretty much the only non–fully white person in a predominantly Caucasian town). And depending on the time in my life, I either felt too skinny or too fat. Like many women, I suffered when I thought about my looks. But suffering isn't always bad. It can be an impetus for all of us to seek deeper and, ultimately, to learn and grow.

Everything about beauty in the mainstream sense of the word is about comparison, contrast, and competition. I'm not sure how we got here, but here we are—focusing on division, not harmony. It's often about highlighting differences, which then leads to all the numerous ways of promoting the idea that you are never enough—not thin enough, not fit enough, not pretty enough, not perfect enough, booty not big enough, hair not lush enough.

My perspective of beauty is now very simple: it is okay to work to improve your appearance, have fun with products, express your uniqueness through experimenting with different looks, all of it. It's all fine, so long as you don't mistake any of that for True Beauty.

TRUE BEAUTY

In essence, True Beauty *is* the True Self, so you are already beautiful, by definition, because the True Self is you! **But it is *the degree* to which someone is connected to the True Self inside of them that makes their true beauty shine through.**

When Yogananda says, "Live quietly in the moment and see the beauty of all before you,"[3] he is referring to the formless beauty that runs through all. Including you and me. We get so caught up in form and appearance, but that is a teeny tiny fraction of who we are. And it's not what makes you truly beautiful.

The most powerfully attractive, beautiful people are the ones who are the most comfortable and accepting of themselves. They know the open secret: that they are so much more than the surface. They are in touch and connected with the true essence of who they are underneath, whether they themselves use those words or not. There is a complete naturalness about them, no matter how well-defined their features are or if they wear glittery makeup or not, because they are in harmony with themselves.

The women I now think of when the word *beauty* comes up, women who are so beautiful they literally bring a tear to my eye, include Jane Goodall, Anandamayi Ma, Eleanor Roosevelt, and Maya Angelou. Their sustained beauty that surpasses time and place has nothing to do with what they look like. Sure, you might like checking out some pretty Instagram pics for passing fun, but I would choose timeless, true, and deeper beauty for real life. The kind of beauty that keeps getting deeper and better and more interesting as time goes on, like an evolving garden. Wouldn't you?

True Beauty is *so* different from what we've been told beauty is. True Beauty is formless. It's an energy. You are pure energy, and the beauty inside of you is your energy, your unique expression of life force. You are beautiful because you are you and the unique expression of energy inside of you. Period.

When we are naturally ourselves, we've connected with our True Selves. We are not trying to be something we are not, not trying to talk like or look like someone else. It means we are deeply connected to the essence inside. And that essence is a unique manifestation of the Divine. There is no other manifestation of Spirit quite like you.

You are completely one of a kind. **You are energy and light underneath all the surface stuff that is powerful and wonderful, and is beautiful by definition.** Not for what it looks like, though of course some people have physical beauty, too, and that's great. **You are beautiful regardless of what you look like. You are beautiful because of who you really are.**

Yogananda urges us to follow the path of "wisdom, beauty, and love."[4] He is placing beauty, in this sense, in the same category as wisdom and love! He also speaks of the infinite beauty of Spirit. That is the real beauty, the kind that will fill your heart with so much love that no longer will you berate yourself or your looks, no longer will you complain how stupid or boring or fat you are. For you will finally know that you *are* the beauty of Spirit. You've been trying to "get" beauty all along, like trying to get love or get validation. All along, you just had to look deeper to see that the beauty you've always chased is right here, right now.

SHIFTING FOCUS

When you realize this is the truth of what beauty is, you then start to shift your focus. It happens very naturally, so you don't need to worry about it too much. It's like watching my elder son's interests shift from playing with toy garbage trucks to learning about complex facts on dinosaurs, along with some pretty intense dinosaur species names (like *Pachycephalosaurus* and *Suchomimus*!). There's nothing forced here; it's merely a natural shifting of energy and focus.

When this starts to happen, you will still care about your appearance. But it simply won't take up as much of your time. It will be important to you, but not dire. Instead of endlessly focusing on your appearance, you spend some time on it and then move over to spending more of your time connecting with your true beauty through the True Self. You allow more time for stillness and meditation. Your priorities shift.

How does this look in the real world? I'll use myself as an example. I still wake up, put on very high-quality, high-performance skin care (that I manufacture myself, so yes, I still love and am quite into skin care!), because sure, I want my skin to look as good as possible. On the road to enlightenment, you can still care about preventing fine lines and skin damage. The two are not mutually exclusive. I put on some makeup, though not as much or as often as I used to wear it. Then I pretty quickly move on.

Relaxing about our looks, because we know we are so much more, is one of the signs that we are starting to connect with our True Beauty. Like me, it doesn't mean that you don't care or that you don't want to look hot for your significant other or feel physically beautiful as you walk down the street. But it does mean learning to chill out. Who are we really trying to impress? You know you are more than just the way you look. The Sufi mystic Rumi also gives us all a great reminder (especially us ladies) when he writes, "I am not this hair, I am not this skin, I am the soul that lives within."

Now, you might have trouble accepting this, especially when the world can be so judgmental. But here is a simple truth. The world is always going to judge you. That's what the world, society, other people do. It's part of what makes us human—it's not necessarily something to be proud of, but it is a truth. Someday when we can all attain states of higher living and embrace the True Self, things might be different, but people are sizing you up all the time. It's partly a defense mechanism that goes back hundreds of thousands of years. Are you a potential threat? Are you a potential mate?

Yet constant evaluation of ourselves and others can lead to a great deal of suffering. Stop adding to that chaos and attitude by being kinder to yourself and others and by easing up on your own judgments. I know wounds around our looks can penetrate deeply, but if you focus more on the reality that you are beautiful just as you are— and so is the person across from you and on TV and on the line at the drugstore—your personal acceptance will expand and expand. Here's a way to help you do just that.

Self-Reflection: Seeing Your True Beauty

My Ayurvedic teacher, Vaidya Jay, taught me about the Ayurvedic practice of mirror-gazing as part of one's morning practice, which was mentioned in the ancient text Bhavaprakash. At first, I thought, "How basic! Everyone looks in the mirror every day."

But it's actually not basic. It's a powerful way to connect to your True Beauty. Besides meditation, which I will say for the hundredth time is the singular most powerful way to connect with your True Self, and therefore your True Beauty, this mirror-gazing practice is another practice I recommend for accessing your unique beauty from within the depths of the soul.

You see, when most of us look in the mirror, we may look to see how our hair looks, if we have anything stuck in our teeth, to apply makeup. None of us really gazes deeply into our own eyes, at least not on a regular basis.

Over time, this practice can help you foster self-love. It can bring up a lot, especially at first, when you aren't used to truly looking at yourself. Eventually you will start to connect and feel growing love, growing compassion within you and for you. You may realize that you don't yet know yourself at all, because you've never really connected to the True Self and your True Beauty up until this point. You may be astonished to find the light of your energy is startling to you, and that yes, there really is some intense beauty radiating from inside of you. Yes, you!

Let's get into the practice.

1. **Find a mirror where you can at least see your entire face, and that is comfortable for you to sit in front of pretty closely, say one to two feet away.** You can use a hand-held mirror or pull up a chair or sit on the floor in front of a full-length mirror.

2. **Pull back your hair.** Move your hair out of your eyes, which can often obstruct our faces and our full gaze. Relax your judgment about yourself and any part of your physical appearance.

3. **Start connecting.** Now, start looking deeply into your own eyes. At first, you might find yourself darting back and forth between each of your eyes. That's okay. First, focus on your right eye and take some deep breaths. Try to keep from overly blinking. Remind yourself that you are safe and that you are loved.

   Then shift your focus to your left eye and refocus your gaze there. Take some more deep breaths and allow your body to continue relaxing. Notice any differences in your perspective that come up in the difference between your two eyes. Keep your breathing long and deep and steady. Stay on

this eye for a while, then return to your right eye
and so on.

It can feel confrontational at first, but stay with
it for at least for 2 minutes. Over time you can build
up to 5 or 10 minutes.

- **Really see.** What are you supposed to see? Your
  True Self. The light within. You may be looking at
  yourself for the first time. You may feel vulnerable
  doing this. You may also feel some inklings of
  wounds, pain, and unaddressed emotions that
  start to bubble up (which was the case for me the
  first time I did this). Hold the space for yourself
  and keep reminding yourself that you are safe
  and supported and that you are loved. Also
  remind yourself that you are so much more than
  what you look like. You are so much more than
  the surface.

You might start to feel tremendous compassion for
yourself. You might start to connect to the innocent, kind
being inside of you. You might start to feel self-love, maybe
for the first real time. You may also not really connect too
much at first. That's okay too. Whatever comes up, just
witness it and stay with the practice. If your gaze drops
from your eyes, bring it right back up.

Some Ayurvedic practitioners recommend doing this
practice every morning for at least a moment or two, to
connect with the True Self before you start your day. I recommend trying to do this practice at least once a week or
every other week.

You can also do little check-ins when you look in the
mirror in the morning. For at least a few seconds, look
right in your eyes and try to see your deeper self, and tell
yourself that you love yourself! You love the light within.

PART III

Chapter 15

YOU ARE MAGNETIC

"Why is it that when some people speak,
everyone is enthralled, while others can talk about
the same thing and no one is interested? . . . What is the
secret of this power? It is called magnetism."

— PARAMAHANSA YOGANANDA[1]

YOUR MAGNETIC POTENTIAL

I remember playing with magnets for the first time in Mrs. Robinson's first-grade class. I was astounded to see that you could make another magnet move just by holding another one in your hand at a specific angle. Sometimes a magnet can attract and sometimes they can repel, but what fascinated me was the invisible energy that was doing the moving! It felt like magic, and as I moved the magnets around in my hands, I felt like a magician.

Imagine if you could learn to be like a magnet and draw the things you want into your life. That would mean you wouldn't have to pull or push; you wouldn't have to struggle or stress. You could simply attract good people, helpful circumstances, and golden opportunities to you.

Actually, you don't have to imagine this. Each and every one of us has the ability to draw happiness and prosperity into our lives. It just takes a little practice and understanding to access the natural magnetic potential inside of you. As you learn to develop your own personal magnetism, you'll begin attracting positive things like good fortune, exciting opportunities, and people who will raise you to new levels of experiences.

And with just a little understanding of your personal magnetic quality, you'll also begin to realize how you may be repelling good people and events too—just like that inverted magnet that pushes other magnets away. Yogananda teaches, "By soul magnetism, the spiritual magnetism in man, a person draws to himself friends and desired objects, and acquires profound knowledge."[2]

One of my most dramatic personal examples of being magnetic was how I first connected with Deepak Chopra in person. My third book, *The Beauty Detox Power*, was the point where my writing and my work started to take a definite philosophical, spiritual turn. Deepak had always been a role model to me in the realm of connecting Eastern and Western philosophy. I had read many of his books and thought he was the best possible person to get an endorsement from for this new book.

I sent his team the book, and waited and waited. I stayed positive and followed up, and after months of trying to make contact, I finally heard back from his team that he loved the book and had agreed to give the book an endorsement. I was thrilled, but I also felt that he and I were meant to collaborate even more deeply beyond that. I focused on what that might be like, and as I got really clear on the vision of it (more on how to do that later), I felt great gratitude and joy at the prospect. During this time, I was going deeper and deeper into my practice and self-work, and letting go of old, unprocessed emotions that were weighing me down. I was increasingly feeling lighter and more connected to myself and everything else.

Fast forward a few months. I was living in New York City at the time and was walking to a meeting in Gramercy Park from my apartment in the West Village. I would usually cut through Union Square, which made the most sense because it was the fastest way to my destination. That day, however, for some reason I can't explain, I felt strongly impelled to walk to the west of the park and go around the perimeter. And who do I run into right smack on the sidewalk? Deepak Chopra!

"Deepak, it's me, Kimberly! You just reviewed my book!" I blurted out in my excitement. Though we had never met in person, Deepak was incredibly warm. The encounter felt as joyful as I had imagined. We chatted, and that single conversation led to collaborating on videos and other content. Eventually we co-authored a book together called *Radical Beauty*. If I ever doubted the existence of magnetism, I never did again after that day.

HOW TO BE A MAGNET

So how do you access the magnetic quality that is part of your True Self? Your True Self is the embodiment of all the high-vibration emotions. You attract the good things in life through positive, high-vibration emotions like love, joy, kindness, peace, and gratitude. On the flip side, you repel what you want through negative, low-vibration emotions like anger, envy, jealousy, hate, fear, and chronic sadness.

You might say you want an exciting new job, but if the energy you are putting out into the world is sluggish, it can block your dream career from manifesting in your life. Negative, depressed energy repels what you want and in turn can inadvertently draw to you all the people, situations, and things that you *don't* want. Case in point: let's say you want to create a successful business. If you are critical and judgmental of others, your energy literally pushes people away—good managers, staff, and customers. Lower-vibration emotions create energy patterns in your life that keep you small and limited. Like tends to go to like. As Yogananda says, "Those whose thoughts are inharmonious will always find inharmony."[3]

Now I know what you may be thinking. The terms *high vibration* and *low vibration* might remind you of your woo woo–loving friend who always tells you she is sending you "good vibes." Yet there is supportive science that suggests that vibrations play a fundamental role in our lives. Researchers from the University of California, Santa Barbara, have developed a "resonance theory of consciousness," with is based on data from the fields of neuroscience, biology, and physics.[4] This theory suggests that resonance—which is another word for "being in sync"—is at the heart of not only human consciousness but of physical reality in general.[5]

In science the phenomenon of "spontaneous self-organization" refers to when frequencies start synchronizing. In his book *Sync: How Order Emerges from Chaos in the Universe, Nature, and Daily Life,* Steven Strogatz provides various examples from physics, biology, chemistry, and neuroscience to illustrate what he calls "sync" (synchrony), where frequencies start matching up.[6] One example is how large gatherings of fireflies of certain species start flashing in sync with one another (it reminds me of flash mobs—groups of diverse people coming together in a public place to dance to something fun, like a Prince song).[7]

Research from the HeartMath Institute, which is based on different physiological tests such as EEG (brain waves), SCL (skin conductance), ECG (heart), BP (blood pressure), hormone levels, and heart rate variability, has found that stressful or depleting emotions such as frustration and overwhelm lead to disorder that is reflected throughout virtually all bodily systems.[8]

So how does this relate to personal magnetism? Well, emotions have frequencies. You can tune in to how certain emotions feel to you in your own body. You'll find that when you are experiencing states of love and joy, you feel "lighter," which is indicative of a higher vibration. When you feel negative emotions, let's say anger or hate, those feelings in your body will feel quite dense, which are indicative of lower vibrations. The work of David R. Hawkins, M.D., Ph.D., the psychiatrist we mentioned in Chapter 12, attempts to apply measurable scientific analysis to our emotions.

Hawkins developed what he called the "Scale of Consciousness," which uses a muscle-testing technique called Applied Kinesiology.[9] Essentially, this alternative medicine practice measures your body's response to emotions and gives each emotion a number on a scale. Peace, joy, and love rank highest, while fear, apathy, guilt, and shame fall in the gutter. Happiness and fulfillment happen when we are living primarily with the emotions on the highest end of the scale.

Now, this doesn't mean you shouldn't ever feel those low or negative emotions. As humans, we are meant to experience ups and downs, but you want to find a balance, and we do this by feeling our emotions, processing them, and then letting them go. It's like healthy emotional digestion.

Research supports Hawkins's work, and that coherent states of being, characterized by joy, peace, compassion, and gratitude, support the brain and nervous system's ability to function properly and positively influence your perceptions, emotions, intuition, and health. In other words, when your body and brain work better and more cohesively, you feel better and you perform better.[10]

According to the HeartMath Institute, the way to have more sustained periods of coherence is by "actively self-generating positive emotions."[11] And the way to generate more joy and peace and compassion in an authentic, sustainable way is through a consistent meditation practice! So you can see how all of this starts to go together.

You may be used to wondering, "Why are you so happy today?" when you see a really happy person. "Maybe they just won the lottery or they just got engaged," you tell yourself. We're so conditioned to think that happy, joyful energy results from something outside of oneself. But "self-generated" high-vibration emotions really come from inside of you. And instead of relying on a new purse or a compliment or a raise at work to generate those emotions within you, you start to realize that you can generate them with nothing else besides yourself! And following your meditation techniques, that is.

I offer some exercises here to help you to energize your magnetic capabilities.

Magnetism Manifestation Practice

You can do this practice before going into a situation where you want to be particularly magnetic. It could be a party, a meeting, a dinner date, an interview, or whatever. This will help put you into the highest possible vibrational state, so that you can exude that powerful force that will help you attract what you want in your life.

It takes as little as a few minutes, yet it is a powerful tool in your toolbox. I often do this practice before recording podcasts.

1. To start, shake out your hands, your body, and/or your head a few times. Imagine that you are shaking off any negative thoughts, negative energy, the heaviness of the day, or anything that might have happened earlier that annoyed or worried you.

2. Next, close your eyes and take some deep breaths, for a few moments at least. As you watch the breath, notice how it starts to slow down.

3. Now, put all your attention on your heart. Focus on three words: *Love, Peace, Joy.* Feel these emotions in your heart. Use your will, as Yogananda teaches us, to direct energy into your heart, and self-generate these emotions until you actually feel their presence. You might feel disconnected from these emotions in your own life. If so, think of a scene in a happy (even if it's cheesy) movie where the characters embodied these emotions, and work with that.

    Once you call those emotions into your heart, imagine they are spreading out from your heart in all directions, to all the cells of your body, like a dam that bursts open and allows the river to flow freely. Feel the warmth of these emotions as they saturate you. I like to imagine it as a warm white light.

4.   Once you feel completely saturated in these high-vibration emotions, close your hands in prayer, bring them to your chest, and take a moment for gratitude. Acknowledge the good in your life, and anything specific that comes up for you. Gratitude is a high-vibration state, so it will also amplify your magnetism.

Okay, now you're ready! Go for it. Now you're in your highest vibe state to rock it (whatever it is that you want to rock).

FREEDOM

Great saints and yogis were so magnetic that followers sought them out. For instance, the great Kriya Yoga master Lahiri Mahasaya returned to his home in Varanasi after receiving Kriya Yoga for the first time from the great yogi Babaji in a forest. He was trying to live a quiet life, but crowds started to gather around him with no effort or intention on his part. Yogananda wrote in *Autobiography of a Yogi*, "As the fragrance of flowers cannot be suppressed, so Lahiri Mahasaya, quietly living as an ideal householder, could not hide his innate glory. Devotee-bees from every part of India began to seek the divine nectar of the liberated master."[12]

Notice how in the above quote Yogananda refers to the great saint as a "liberated master." As you work toward your own liberation, your freedom, your ability to be magnetic becomes more powerful. You liberate yourself from feeling small and fearful and limited. And then you become like a beacon of light, through which the rays of freedom shine, illuminating a path for others, and drawing people and opportunities to you naturally and powerfully.

Other Practical Ways to Become More Magnetic in Your Life

1. **Speak only from your soul.** Yogananda taught that if you speak with the full power of your soul behind your words, people will want to listen and will draw closer to hear you. This means to speak with sincerity, humility, passion. Speak right from your heart.

   One of the reasons I think my husband, Jon, is so magnetic and that people often flock to listen to what he has to say is that he is entirely authentic. When he speaks, it is truth, and he never tries to hide anything. It's powerful, and in that kind of free energy, others can relax as themselves. On a recent birthday I held a circle (like the kind I mentioned in Chapter 6, YOU ARE WHOLE) for some of our friends, and when people went around to say some words about Jon, most everyone mentioned his authenticity and his integrity.

   People do notice your speech and the way you conduct yourself. Speak your truth from a connected place deep inside of you and with kindness and compassion as well, and you will be even more magnetic.

2. **Listen well.** Listen most of the time and speak only when you have something you really want

to share, and not just to fill silence or talk out of nervous habit. We mentioned this briefly in Chapter 12 as it relates to being a powerhouse, and it's also relevant here: talking too much can actually diminish your magnetism. It burns a lot of your energy to talk all the time, and besides, idle chatter is usually pretty shallow. Save your words for when you really have something to say, and that way when do you speak, your words will be laden with meaning and power.

3. **Look within.** Self-awareness is a very important aspect of this path. Many of our chapters include reflections so you can look at how these teachings apply to your own life. You must continue to analyze yourself on a daily basis so you can stop living out old, unconscious patterns and reactions and start walking in your truth. Nothing is more magnetic than someone who walks their walk.

4. **Use your will to create.** Yogananda taught that when you use your will to create in the world, whatever is your focus, you are developing your magnetism. This is because the more you use your will, the more you are directing prana, or life force, to command your will. More will equals more energy, which is by nature more magnetic. Think about this: Are you more drawn to someone who is alive and trying to accomplish something in the world, or someone who is a couch potato and can only recommend to you which shows to binge on? We both know that answer.

5. **Integrate magnetism from saints and other great ones.** Yogananda taught that when you meditate and pray, you should feel that saints or other spiritual figures or people that you admire and connect with are with you. And that you can integrate some of their magnetism into your life. This can also include inspiring, non-saint people, too, such as Justice Ruth Ginsburg, your grandmother, Harriet Tubman, Martin Luther King Jr., Ralph Waldo Emerson, and so on.

    Try creating a little meditation space or a sort of altar or focus point in your home where you gather special objects that have great meaning for you. Be sure to include some photos of those people who greatly inspire you to give yourself a visual reference point. My space has photos of Yogananda and the rest of the Kriya Yoga yogis, Jesus, and statues of Buddha. There's no shortage of magnetism inspiration going on at home!

6. **Create the right environment.** The environment that you surround yourself with is of critical importance, for it will influence your energy and your magnetism. Yogananda urged us to be around positive people, people who are calm and in control of themselves and exemplify other qualities that you admire. It can also be helpful to seek out and attune to the energy of those who have integrity and are successful in the field you would like to succeed in. On the other hand, avoid those who leave you feeling depleted or negative or simply down in some

way. Be discerning with who you surround yourself with, always!

Sometimes I've had to figure out how to carefully and very kindly avoid being around certain people. I try to do this lovingly, reminding myself that in protecting my energy, I'm able to serve more in the world.

7. **Stick to a lifestyle that supports your goals.** On a practical level, you need to maintain your living habits in a way that enables you to protect the vital forces in your body. For instance, overloading the body by overeating diminishes your life force and your magnetism. So be sure to eat only as much as you need to, sticking mostly to lighter, easily digested plant foods. Don't overtax your body with drugs and alcohol. If you don't pay attention, it's easy sometimes to let the after-work wine or other drinks start to creep up. Be your own personal manager over your lifestyle and make the adjustments necessary when anything feels imbalanced.

Chapter 16

PRACTICE:
How to Effectively
Do Affirmations

*"Words saturated with sincerity, conviction,
faith, and intuition are like highly explosive vibration
bombs, which, when set off, shatter the rocks of
difficulties and create the change desired."*

— PARAMAHANSA YOGANANDA[1]

THE POWER OF YOUR WORDS

Understanding that we are all powerful creators is one of the fundamental principles of Yogananda's teachings. The True Self is always creating. And one of the easiest and most effective ways of directing this energy is through the power of the words you use.

With a world population nearing 8 billion people, words are more copious today than they ever have been. Millions of conversations are happening right now, everywhere around the globe. There are more books, magazines, and movies being produced than ever before. And the internet? Well, there may well be an infinite number of words—good and bad—being used there that contribute exponentially to a never-ending cycle. And unfortunately, with all of this chatter that goes on minute by minute and day by day, it is impossible to comprehend all the words flying at us. It then devolves into a lot of noise and starts to feel like the *blah blah blah* sounds of listening to Charlie Brown's teacher.

The phrase *talk is cheap* is one all of us have heard at one time or another. While it usually means, "I won't believe what you're saying until you give me proof," it also suggests that words have lost their value in many ways. We speak idly, we fill empty spaces with words, we go off into unfocused conversations and just chat away without really thinking too much about what we are saying.

Yet words have awesome, creative power, especially when used consciously and directed toward a goal. "I love you," "We will succeed," "Never give up": these words contain strength and beauty that inspire us and help us grow. And yet, like any creative power, words are a double-edged sword—they can build up or tear down. Most of us unknowingly take this for granted, otherwise why would we so casually declare, "I'm such a loser," "I'm so gross and fat," "There are no good men/women left for me," or "This is all such a nightmare, and it's never going to work out."

Words help to create your day-to-day reality. I've never met a successful person who repeatedly denigrates herself. In fact, when you use negative self-talk, you are sowing the seeds of turmoil and hardship. Bottom line: you speak into existence the words that you think and say.

WORD MYTHS

The idea of affirmations has been floating around in self-help circles for over a hundred years. And unfortunately, they have gotten a bad rap because of the ineffectual way they are often used—casual and not fully directed.

If you just sit around and say things like "I'm rich!" with no feeling or focused intention, then affirmations are a waste of time. In the end, you're just lying to yourself. No one around you believes it, certainly not you, and most importantly, your lukewarm attempt at expanding your life fizzles and goes cold.

Most of us haven't been taught how to really perform affirmations to their fullest, most powerful form. So, when they fail, we cast away affirmations like old socks that don't really fit us, and in the process unknowingly cast away a potentially incredibly effective technique that you can use to manifest what you want.

THE POWER OF PROPERLY PRACTICED AFFIRMATIONS

Yogananda had a lot to say about the power of doing affirmations properly. He teaches, "That is why all affirmations of the conscious mind should be impressive enough to permeate the subconsciousness, which in turn automatically influences the conscious mind. . . . Still stronger affirmations reach not only the subconscious but also the superconscious mind—the magic storehouse of miraculous powers."[2]

So properly doing affirmations doesn't mean you just rattle off a bunch of phrases. Nor does it mean negating the power of your words by saying, "I am healthy and fit" while thinking, "Yeah, right. This doesn't work. I'm actually the epitome of being out of shape." When you combine words with a committed intention and powerful emotion, you unite that energy with each word you are saying.

The truth of this is wonderfully exemplified by my friend Dan Buettner, National Geographic Fellow and founder of the Blue Zones, which is an organization that teaches communities how to emulate the five regions in the world where people live much longer than usual. I asked him if he uses affirmations in his conquests, and he recounted:

In a moment of rapture, or perhaps too much tequila, I declared to a few friends that I was going to bike across Africa— an affirmation of sorts. I started researching the trip: crossing the Sahara, traveling parallel to the equator through the Congo, then to the top of Mt. Kilimanjaro, the Serengeti, and down to Cape Town. And I got very excited. I told more and more people about it and got them excited. Pretty soon, I got three teammates excited—and 15 sponsors. Finally, we were dipping our rear wheels in the sea north of Tunisia to begin the trip.

But the story doesn't end here. Two thousand one hundred miles into the Sahara, the road ended, and we faced raw, open desert. The easy thing would have been to retreat. Instead, we pushed on. In the Congo, we found almost no food. We contracted malaria, dysentery, intestinal worms, and giardiasis. We were emaciated, filthy, and defeated. What kept us going? That same declaration that got me started. But now, it had taken on a different type of power. I had made promises to sponsors who counted on us and friends who believed in us.

What had started as an affirmation had now transformed into a resolve not to let people down. And you know what? It pushed us through. On June 10, 1993, after 12,220 miles, we rolled into Cape Town, South Africa, and set the Guinness World Record for cycling Africa. The lesson: Beware of what you declare during a time of rapture.

Bottom line: affirmation plus willpower leads to transformation. So don't just recite your affirmations; really live them.

Yogananda was a pioneer in the science of affirmation and began teaching the technique long before it became a modern-day practice. Here is some guidance he gives: "Choose your affirmation and repeat all of it, first loudly, then softly and more slowly, until your voice becomes a whisper. Then gradually affirm it mentally only, without moving the tongue or the lips, until you feel that you have attained deep, unbroken concentration—not unconsciousness, but a profound continuity of uninterrupted thought. If you continue with your mental affirmation, and go still deeper, you will feel a sense of increasing joy and peace. During the state of deep concentration, your affirmation will merge with the subconscious stream, to come back later reinforced with power to influence your conscious mind through the law of habit."[3]

This is what happened to my friend Dan. He had embedded his affirmation so deeply inside himself that it began to manifest and influence the decisions he made. Coupled with his will to not renege on his affirmation, he attained his dream. And you can do the same.

Here's a simple way to get started:

1. **First of all, create a clear affirmation.**

    It can be one or a few sentences, but you should be able to repeat it from memory. Align with your deepest desire that you find to be fully worthy and aligned with your time and attention. I recommend starting with "I am" to tie in the quality of beingness. Say it in the present tense, to enforce that it's here now, or in the process of coming in. Here are some examples:

    I am passionate about my job, which is fulfilling and meaningful to me.

    I am love, and I find the matching love of my life.

    I am peaceful.

    I am the regional manager. I have a wonderful team to manage.

    I am the owner of my own fashion brand.

2. **Second, repeat the affirmation out loud, then softer and softer, then to a whisper, and finally silently.**

    This means you are ideally going to be saying your affirmation 8–10 times in a session. Keep repeating it within yourself, until you feel that you have attained a deep state of concentration with the words you are saying. As Yogananda says, it should feel like a "profound continuity of uninterrupted thought."[4]

    You need to keep merging with the words you are saying by accepting them as truth. It is important to turn off the tendency to rattle off the words mindlessly, or as Yogananda says, as "blind repetition of demands." This technique requires intense concentration and focus, so it is important to keep your mind on your intention and not on something else, like what you are going to cook for dinner later or a deadline you have to meet.

3. **Remember that this is a practice.**

While seemingly simple, truly merging with your affirmation takes practice.

As I've already mentioned, it's impossible to practice this technique properly if your mind is racing, if you are right in the middle of screaming toddlers, or if you're answering a bunch of texts or playing the news in the background. Instead, it's better to do your affirmations after you meditate, or at least after you put your phone in airplane mode. Once you do, take some deep breaths, and go into a quiet space. Otherwise, just wait for the right opportunity, because if you do it without the concentration required, you are just wasting your time.

4. **Look for peace as a marker for effectiveness.**

Yogananda teaches that if we find ourselves going into deeper and deeper states, we are indeed allowing the affirmation to go deeper and deeper into our "superconscious realm, to return later laden with unlimited power to influence your conscious mind and also to fulfill your desires."[5]

Feelings of increasing peace are a definite marker that you are going deeper into the affirmation and uniting with it, so that it will manifest as your reality in your life. Feel that the affirmation is becoming part of you, actually merging into your heart and then through every cell and part of you.

5. **Move on and believe.**

Once you complete the practice, which can take anywhere from, say, three minutes or so to as much time as you want to stay in that state, be convinced that your affirmation has been heard and that what is Spirit's is also yours. Then move on with your day with that confidence and knowing.

You can make affirmations part of your daily life and daily practice. Or you can weave them in and out as you feel connected to using them. There isn't a "right" timing and frequency. If you are really focused on a goal, though, I suggest you practice them daily. Try them, wield your own power, and create away!

Note: if you are looking for affirmation inspiration, Paramahansa Yogananda offers hundreds of affirmations for healing, self-improvement, and deepening your unity with the True Self in the *Self-Realization Fellowship Lessons* and the books *Scientific Healing Affirmations* and *Metaphysical Meditations*.

Chapter 17

YOU ARE ABUNDANCE

*"If man works in harmony with the divine
law of success, he receives abundance. . . ."*

— PARAMAHANSA YOGANANDA[1]

OUR ABUNDANT NATURE

I grew up in New England, and in the fall, my family would drive to Vermont to see the beautiful changing leaves. When I peered out the window from the backseat of the car, I was astounded by the mountains covered by thousands of trees sporting gorgeous red, gold, orange, and purple leaves. Years later, I visited a remote area of the Philippines and had a similar experience. As I looked out the car window, I was struck by the coconut trees that stretched for miles and miles. There were zillions of them! Both times I felt awed by the grandeur—and the abundance—of the world around me.

If you stop for a moment, look around, and take in your surroundings, you'll see that abundance is all around us, not just in the trees, but *everywhere*. Visit the produce section of a supermarket, observe the endless miles of streets and roads that connect us to each other, dive into an ocean teeming with life, breathe in the air around you, count the grains of sand in the desert, consider the trillions of dollars that sit in banks all over the world, or imagine the names of the more than 7 billion people who are our brothers and sisters in this human race.

Or just consider you. Think of the abundance of plenty that makes up your body. You have over a billion cells in your body, and each cell is performing its own function and is simultaneously working together as a whole. You have 79 organs in your body. You have more than 600 muscles. You have on average 5 liters of blood in your circulatory system. You can talk, walk, dance, and sing, and even if you don't do these things well, you still can move and think and argue and make love.

Abundance is a state of plenty. It is prosperity in all its forms, not just money, but love, friendships, resources, opportunities, and so on. It is the very nature of the True Self, which is always giving and giving. And this means that you are abundance as well.

To live as abundance and in abundance, we need to have an abundance mindset, which means becoming aware of the inherent creative life force *within* us. Perhaps you may feel like there's scarcity in your life right now— maybe you don't have all the money or the love that you want. But when you learn to turn on your abundance mindset, which is what this chapter is all about, you will discover that you can have your share of all you desire.

Though abundance is all around us, we still live in a world of need and want. That's one of the tragedies of life. Abundance is our birthright, yet many people lack even the basic necessities of food, water, shelter, companionship, and love. Yet, in developing an abundance mindset, you'll realize that there is plenty for you to cultivate and give to those around you. True abundance is about expanded thinking, the realization that you can have what you want and that you can also help others in need.

BELIEVING IS SEEING

Of course, embracing abundance can be difficult. If you're like most people, you'll believe something when you see it. You don't have a lot of time for flighty theories or wishful thinking (especially if, unlike all of those zillions of coconut trees I referenced earlier, the area where you live has only a few straggly trees in a local park). You want evidence. And evidence may take on very different forms, including reviews for a potential dentist, compliments that reaffirm how you feel about yourself physically, stats and probabilities of getting pregnant at certain times of your cycle, or sales numbers to predict future sales.

I get it. I used to think I needed to *see something to believe it*. Makes perfect sense. We need facts to build foundations. Facts are like bricks—sturdy and strong. However, it's what we do with the bricks that makes all the difference. We can hurl one into someone's window and cause destruction, or we can construct a beautiful temple of sacred space that reaches high into the sky.

But facts and physical evidence aren't everything. Once I started my meditation practices, it became clear that another rule can be equally important. Namely:

When I believe it, I'll see it.

ABUNDANCE NEEDS SPACE TO GROW

Believe and see. This might sound and feel trippy to you because it propels you into the unknown, which can feel dark and scary. It's hard to cling to anything when you can't see in front of you.

But the dark—the unknown—is the space of pure potentiality. It's the blank canvas that gives rise to all creation and creative ideas you want to manifest. This unlimited space to create, which is always available to you, is the space for abundance—drawing in all that you want in droves, whether it is love, resources, beautiful relationships, or health. The universe, created by Spirit, by definition has no limitations. Whatever you want is there in spades, and there is more than enough to go around.

Think about a beautiful rose. Before it became a rose, seeds had been planted into the soil, into a place of darkness. From there, the seeds were able to gather energy and nutrients and fulfill their potential of blossoming and emerging out of the dark into their beautiful, full form. Every time we close our eyes and meditate, we enter a darkness that can help us grow in new ways too.

CREATING AN ABUNDANCE MINDSET

As I already mentioned, abundance is a quality of the True Self. It comes from inside of you. When most people think of abundance, they longingly look outward and think about all the things they currently don't have and want to pull into them. Things like more money, a soul mate to start a family with or travel with, a more spacious house, a bigger yard, designer clothes.

Yet when we look outward and focus on all the things we don't have, this often leads to feelings of being incomplete, and we feel frustration, and perhaps desperation and despair, when we try to yank things in harder and harder if they aren't coming in the time frame we want. Unfortunately, whether we realize it or not, that creates a lack-based sort of energy that keeps the very things that we want away from us. It's like when the salesperson at the store is so desperate to make a sale and get a commission, she follows you around and keeps pushing the shoes. Finally, you decide you have to escape as soon as possible and run out of the store, whether you want the shoes or not! You didn't get your shoes, and the salesperson didn't get the sale.

Everything is energy, so if we fill ourselves with the energy of missing, not having, and not enough, that is more of what we will get. The more you say you want something, the more you reinforce the belief that you *want* it but don't have it. I know, at first it seems a bit counterintuitive! It's a real shift, though, when you get this.

The best way to create real abundance is to focus on your inner state. This means to feel and focus on cultivating and connecting to the energy of abundance and fullness rising and radiating out from inside of you. **To start creating abundance, focus on the energy you are giving out at this moment, versus what is or isn't coming in right now. You do that by observing if your thoughts or actions are based on fear of not having enough or trust that all will be provided to you.**

I know it can be challenging if you are in a rough patch, living month to month and struggling to pay your rent, or picking which one of the numerous bills that may be piling up to pay right now. Yet you can shift your life.

You *can* lift yourself up and out from where you are, from inside of you. It may feel like a big shift, and maybe you can think of a million reasons why that isn't possible—the job market is crappy, it's too expensive to travel to your dream destination of Tanzania, there just is too much competition in your field.

But you have to go beyond that kind of thinking, even if that's the way you—and everyone surrounding you—currently sees the world. That may be what's showing up now, but there's a whole other system of thinking and a whole new way of living you can tap into that can massively change the state of where you currently are. To access these possibilities, you need to use your will to see beyond the here and now.

Being in an inner state of abundance means that you feel plentiful *now*, that you have trust for life, and that you have faith that more is coming in. And that it will come in its own Divine timing, not the timelines dictated by the often-impatient ego. You believe in the infinite amount of, well, everything! This is the law of abundance, and it's yours to claim right now, no matter what your life currently looks like.

Yogananda illustrates it beautifully in this passage from *Where There Is Light*[2]:

> *Think of Divine Abundance as a mighty, refreshing rain; whatever receptacle you have at hand will receive it. If you hold up a tin cup, you will receive only that quantity. If you hold up a bowl, that will be filled. What kind of receptacle are you holding up to Divine Abundance?*

ABUNDANCE IS RIGHT HERE, RIGHT NOW

Abundance is in the present moment. It definitely does not come from looking to the future, where overthinking only leads to anxiety about how things will work out. This just feeds into lack energy, the exact opposite of abundance! And it also definitely doesn't come from looking back to the past, which can be overevaluated and can create fear about the future. It has to be in the here and now.

If you start to purposely create an inner state of abundance, if you focus on all the richness in you and around you, your outer world will eventually have to match that inner energy. And then, without the desperation of trying over and over again to pull things in, you do. It just happens.

Focusing on your inner state, feeling full and plentiful, along with trust and faith, will also create an easeful state of flow in your life. Opportunities, amazing friendships and connections, and customers will start coming in. It doesn't mean there's no effort, because you can't just walk around in your pajamas all day watching YouTube and then lament that no one is chasing you for work.

But it does mean the end of *over*-efforting. As well as the end of excessive stress and worry. So this means monitoring your thoughts from moment to moment. Where are you on the scale of abundance in each "now" moment? Do you feel plentiful, or do you feel lack?

I must admit I used to be skeptical about this concept. But then I put Yogananda's words into action. Los Angeles is a notoriously competitive real estate environment. When we were ready to buy our dream house, we fell in love with a specific location that doesn't have that much inventory—one of the reasons we loved it! It is a little mountain canyon area about 30 minutes outside of the city's edge, which is far enough to feel like a completely different world but still close enough to be part of the greater city's community and resources.

"Reality" was painted to us in terms of horror stories from friends about losing houses left and right to other buyers and having to pay well above the asking price. I absolutely did not want to have to deal with bidding wars, and the last thing I wanted to do was spend countless weekends looking at dozens of houses. Despite the so-called evidence, I declared to my husband, Jon, that there is abundance everywhere and enough for all, and finding our house was going to be super easy. It was a pretty bold declaration because it was contrary to what the market showed. "Okay, babe," Jon said and smiled. I'm not sure he fully believed me, but he also knows better than to try to talk me down from something I feel passionate about.

I kept saying it out loud to myself and to others: it's super easy to find our house! I even said this affirmation after my meditations and felt pure excitement in my body. Inwardly, I just kept focusing on feeling abundant from the inside. And even though the circumstances didn't exactly support it, I stuck to it and kept feeling it.

We looked at one house, which wasn't quite right, then a second. Too much fixing up. Then we looked at a third house. It had a stunning view of the mountains, a flat area with a lawn and gardens and some wild areas, and spanned over nearly an acre, including six redwood trees and several huge oak trees, and over a dozen fruit trees. It was our house! It was more than I imagined, with so much abundance of nature and space and beauty. The second time we saw it, Jon accidentally left his phone in the kitchen. When we came back to get it, we met the owner, Katy. This is never supposed to happen in usual Realtor etiquette!

Yet we were able to make a personal connection with her, and we shared that we were pregnant with another child and were excited for this to be our family house. The ending of the story is that we put in an offer lower than the asking. Katy met us halfway. I can't help but think it made a difference that we got to meet her. We went into escrow, at which time several other buyers also became interested. But we were locked in and closed in 45 days. We got our dream house in a pretty much "super easy" way, just as I had declared from an abundance mindset.

The Abundance State Practice

Try doing this throughout the day as often and as much as you can. You can do this practice in the quiet moments while working, playing with your children, cooking, cleaning out your garage, anytime. It eventually becomes a living practice that you don't have to stop and do, but something you live.

1. To start, it can help to close your eyes and pause to tune in. No matter what is going on outside of you, sense your inner state. Maybe you feel a bit empty at that moment, or maybe you're starting in a place where you already feel big energy.

2. Now start to consciously create a state of abundance like stoking a fire. How do you do that? You focus on it. You can self-generate the feelings of expansion, fullness, prosperity, and plenty. Use your will and create them inside of yourself.

You don't have to think of specific things in this practice unless you feel called to or if it initially helps you tap into the feelings. I just like to focus on generating the pure feeling of abundance—that there is plenty of everything—and feeling open, which can attract any number of things. Including things that Spirit has in store for us that we can't even think of yet.

Self-generate the feeling for at least two to three minutes with your full focus.

3. Try to hold on to that feeling of abundance for as long as you can. Keep this mindset even as you open your eyes and keep going about your day. The abundant feeling usually comes and goes for almost all of us, until that full enlightenment stage where it is our total way of living. But for now, let's keep it real. We're all human, and so the realization is going to flicker a bit. That's okay! Just keep going in and checking in often to your inner state, and have faith that the more you feel abundant, the more that repeated vibration must start to match in your outside world.

THE ABUNDANCE-GRATITUDE CONNECTION

Gratitude is a potent energy because it supports your abundance mindset. When you are grateful, you look around at all the amazing things around you, all your infinite gifts. It connects you to abundance energy. And so it allows more goodness to flow in.

When I interviewed Matthew and Terces Engelhart, the founders of the vegan chain Café Gratitude, for my podcast, I asked them about their business's spectacular growth. At their height, they had over 700 employees. They recalled how when they were starting out, their first cafe was often empty. But despite that, they focused on feeling supremely grateful for every single dollar that came in, and for every customer who gave them a shot. As their café name so aptly reflects, gratitude became a dominant daily force in their lives, and from that energy of appreciation they were able to keep growing and create thriving success.

If, however, you keep rushing around from one thing to the next and don't even pause to be grateful for what you *do* have, you can shut out great things from coming your way. Why? Because you aren't connecting to the energy of abundance. I've met people, and you probably have, too, who have a lot of things, like financial wealth, a wonderful family, great friends, and so on. But still, they aren't abundant. They don't take in what is there, and they aren't grateful. So instead, they sit in lack energy. They are ever looking outward at the next thing they "need" to be happy because they sure aren't happy in this present moment. Sadly, they never connect to true happiness and true contentment. They remain restless and in the state of never feeling like they are enough or like they have enough.

You don't want to be one of those people! Yogananda's wisdom teaches us, "If a drunken prince goes into the slums and, forgetting entirely his true identity, begins lamenting, 'How poor I am,' his friends will laugh at him and say, 'Wake up, and remember that you are a prince.'"[3]

Self-Reflection: Gratitude Now

Take a pause and whip out your journal. Just start listing all the things you are grateful for. Notice that even if your life right now is not where you want it to be, there is still an enormous list of things to be grateful for, from having a bed or a couch to sleep on, toilet paper (most of the world doesn't, as I quickly discovered traveling), stars, sunlight, friendships, your mighty feet for carrying you through each day, your ability to have hopes and dreams, and countless other things.

Tune in and notice how much amazing-ness is truly in your life! If you get into a rut and start feeling in lack, take out your journal and survey your list. And feel free to create new lists regularly, as I do. I love this practice because while our minds can play with us and lead us to believe in lack and the feeling that there's really not enough, this practice is a way to see with our own eyes that abundance is all around and then connect with it in a concrete way.

DARE TO IMAGINE

Also, allowing abundance in any form to come forth—deep, outrageously satisfying love in relationships, ongoing prosperity, perfect health, living your dreams every day—is to imagine that it is even possible in the first place. You need to believe something inside—in your mind, in your heart, in your soul—before you can see it manifest in your outer reality.

A team of researchers from Harvard split in half a group of volunteers who had never played the piano before. One half practiced some simple finger exercises for two hours a day for five days. The other half didn't move their fingers or do the exercise—they just imagined they were sitting at the piano. The before and after brain scans show that both groups created numerous new neural circuits and new neurological programming in the part of the brain that controls finger movements. Amazing! That means that one group was able to enact change through thought alone.[4] This suggests that you and your mind can start creating changes in your body and your life by thinking about your goal clearly and consistently.

In other words, a highly visual faith can create miracles by tapping into the abundance of possibilities within us. So visualize what you want to create in detail, yet also remain open to all that might show up, as we discussed in Chapter 15. The universe might have much far grander opportunities for you beyond what you yourself can imagine at any given time—and you want to be open and receptive to them!

FAITH AND CONFIDENCE

Your thoughts helped to create your present circumstances, so you can't shift to different, more abundant circumstances unless you first change your thoughts.

Jesus said in Mark 11:24, "Therefore I say unto you, What things soever ye desire, when ye pray, believe that ye receive them, and ye shall have them." The key part of this passage is that we believe *before* we receive. We become clear and define what we want, but we do it before it takes form.

Yogananda would agree. He reinforces this with his teaching, "You must believe in the possibility of what you are praying for."[5] Believing that you will create what you want before you see it show up is crucial to successfully creating anything in your life. It doesn't matter if it's a physical healing, a new relationship, a repaired friendship, a new car, a vacation, or even some extra cash to pay off a bill. If you don't really believe it is possible, there will be very different energy as you go about your efforts. If you bring in doubt, you will be met with doubtful outcomes.

Now you might say, sure, I can believe, but what about all the big challenges I might run into? Well, they will still be there. Just because you believe it doesn't mean the path to get to your destination is a perfectly paved, clear path ahead. Bumps and roadblocks are part of any endeavor.

But don't let that intimidate you, even for a minute. Your will is the force that can metaphorically ignite dynamite and clear away those roadblocks. You are so supported because you have the strength and resourcefulness already inside of you. This doesn't necessarily mean that you can do everything on your own. But when you live from a place of faith and abundance, the right people, the right situations, the right advice, help, and support will show up to help you. And you will see that abundance, not lack, is your true natural state.

Practical Steps for Abundant Living

1. **Check in with your moment-to-moment abundance mindset.** Consistently keep checking in to notice if you are in lack or saturating yourself with abundance energy. Do the Abundant State Practice as much as you need until it becomes your primary state of being.

2. **Stay grateful.** Remember that the more you are thankful, the more you connect to abundance and let more amazing things in. So be grateful as much as you can and as often as you can, for all things big and small, and then watch what happens to your prosperity.

3. **Banish doubt.** Don't be discouraged or doubt if something you want doesn't come to pass. Make adjustments if necessary, but stay the course with a firm belief that your abundance is working through you. Sometimes higher intelligence has bigger plans for you, and ultimately things may even work out better than imagined. Keep your focus.

4. **Gain more confidence by small actions.** BJ Fogg, the founder and director of the Behavior Design Lab at Stanford, found that breaking down larger goals into smaller "bite-size" action steps can create dramatic shifts that last.[6] Take smaller steps, like doing some research or reading a book to help build and strengthen your purpose. Then use what you learned to keep moving forward to build more confidence. Anyone who has ever seen an infant take her first steps knows there is a lot of courage involved in getting up and moving in a new way. That baby isn't leaping but taking small steps, and in taking those steps, building strength, focus, and trust. We can learn a lot from little ones.

Chapter 18

PRACTICE:
Working with Mantra

"After acquiring inward treasure, you will find that outward supply is always forthcoming."

— LAHIRI MAHASAYA, AUTOBIOGRAPHY OF A YOGI[1]

What is a mantra, and why is it important? In Sanskrit, *mantra* translates to "instrument or tool of the mind." Mantras are sacred sounds in the form of words, syllables, sayings, prayers, or hymns. They are tools we use to communicate more effectively with the True Self.

Our minds, left to their own devices, have a tendency to run rampant! They are like unruly horses that need to be reined in for their own benefit and for the benefit of others who could get trampled in various circumstances. One of the most important tools at our disposal is the mantra, which can help us focus our minds and help to quiet all that noisy chatter that goes on in between our two ears.

Yogananda taught that "Sound or vibration is the most powerful force in the universe."[2] He promoted the use of mantras both in preliminary meditation techniques and in chanting or devotional music. He even created a whole book of chants in which he teaches, "Music is a divine art, to be used not only for pleasure but as a path to God-realization. Vibrations resulting from devotional singing lead to attunement with the Cosmic Vibration or the Word."[3]

Japa is an ancient yogic practice from Vedic times in which a mantra or the name of a deity is recited repeatedly, either out loud or silently. The practice of japa can be the repetition of a one-word mantra or a mantra made up of a string of words. It comes from the Sanskrit word for "practice," *abhyasa,* which means "repetition." Through our daily practice and repeating these techniques and meditations, we can focus our minds and energy. Japa is usually thought of as an Eastern practice used in Hinduism, Buddhism, Jainism, and Sikhism, but it's also used in Christianity, as evidenced by the use of rosaries, and in Islam and Judaism.

In Yogananda's and other yogic chants, you will find the practice of japa, or in other words, a lot of repetition. It's kind of like when the chorus of a song you get obsessed with gets stuck in your head, and you hum the same line over and over again. That's what japa mantra is like! It's easy to learn, because you say the same words over and over. Yogananda says, "Gradually the subconscious repetition will change into superconscious realization, bringing the actual perception of God. One must chant deeper and deeper until the chanting changes into subconscious and then superconscious realization, bringing one into the Divine Presence."[4]

To get the real use of this tool, though, in the way of deeper realizations and quieting your mind, you have to focus your energy with your will. This was something that Yogananda emphasized time and time again! If you intend to feel peace when you are repeating the word *peace* as your mantra, with deep concentration, you can start to make progress. But if you rattle off a mantra while thinking about which purse you might wear out later to dinner or about a text you have to write, then your words are sadly pretty useless.

Whatever you are doing, put your whole focus into it, including your mantra and meditation practice. In *Star Wars*, Yoda urges Luke to concentrate more and more deeply on using the Force. Once he focused, his aim was mighty and on point. In the same vein, Yogananda states, "Do you know why some people are never able to acquire health or make money, no matter how hard they seem to try? First of all, most people do everything half-heartedly. They use only about one-tenth of their attention."[5] We can do better than one-tenth! You are more, and you'll be able to create your dreams, and higher states of peace and joy, by using more of your attention.

Here are some tips for working with mantras:

1. **Choose the mantra around your intention.**
    For your daily meditation, you might choose the word *Peace*, or *Shanti,* the Sanskrit word for "peace." Or you might choose *Joy, Love, Faith,* or another word that aligns with your intention.

    You can also start working with mantras for other instances, like getting past a difficult time or wanting to manifest something.

    For instance, when we were ready to get pregnant, Jon and I chanted a special, more involved mantra for a healthy conception and pregnancy together, given to me by my Ayurvedic teacher, which I share in our online

Solluna pregnancy course. It surely worked with our intention behind it, and Moses is here with us today!

2. **Say the mantra with increasing concentration and repetition.** Similarly, as with affirmations, mantras are empowered by your focus, devotion, and conviction. As I've said earlier, you need to believe it before you see it. Make sure you dig deep to bring forth your concentration while saying your mantras.

   Say them repeatedly, starting out loud and increasingly quieter into a whisper and then silently, or simply silently the whole time. Remember that repetition builds energy, so keep repeating them over and over again to build real power behind your words!

3. **Bring mantras into your life with music.** If you asked me what I mainly listened to ten years ago, it would have been indie rock. Now, admittedly, mostly what I listen to is kirtan music, which is a kind of call-and-response, mantra-based music. I love the sound and vibration of this type of music, even if I don't understand all the Sanskrit words. It helps me feel even more energized when I listen to it. The "Prema Chalisa," a version of the powerful 108 verse "Hanuman Chalisa," by Krishna Das, played as my wedding song when I walked down the aisle! Besides Krishna Das, some of the other kirtan and chant artists that I love include Wah!, Jai Uttal, Benjy Wertheimer, MC Yogi, The Hanumen, Snatam Kaur, and Deva Premal. Give them a try, or try chanting or

saying mantras alongside other sounds, such as chimes, drums, or crystal bowls.

4. **Here are some other mantras that may resonate with you.** One of Yogananda's ideals in bringing yoga to the West was accessibility, so he did not focus on trying to teach complex, hard-to-pronounce Sanskrit mantras. Still, as a background to yoga, I wanted to offer a few Sanskrit-based mantras to you (and one Buddhist mantra), to help you connect to the original verses, if you are interested. There are infinite mantras, as you can imagine. Here are a few powerful ones, along with a version of their translations:

Aum: the sacred sound of all things. The I AM presence.

Om Namah Shivah: I bow down to the light within. I bow down to the supreme self within.

Hare Krishna: Krishna is the aspect of the Divine that is commonly thought of as love. This mantra was explained to me as, "Everything, everywhere is love."

Aham-Prema: I am Divine love.

Om Mani Padme Hum: This is a Tibetan Buddhist mantra that translates to "Hail the Jewel in the Lotus." It believed to help invoke the ultimate state of compassion, also known as Chenrezig.

Chapter 19

YOU ARE A CREATOR

*"Every human being has some spark of power
by which he can create something that
has not been created before."*

— PARAMAHANSA YOGANANDA[1]

YOU ARE MEANT TO CREATE

Have you ever longed to create something extraordinary in your life? It could be a new idea for an app, a book that teaches kids how to protect the environment, or a new recipe for pairing carrots and chocolate. Maybe you want to start a new website, become a partner at your firm, start your own flower shop, find the love of your life and create a beautiful partnership together, or simply be a wonderful mom or dad.

This desire within you is evidence that you, I, and everyone else is a creator. We want to create things and situations in our lives. When we don't, we feel stagnant, depressed, unfulfilled.

The truth is, you are a creator, and you carry within you the Divine creative spirit that has formed all things.

You were designed to create, and when you work with Spirit on your side, you can sculpt the most amazing life.

Creativity is part of your very DNA, part of your very nature. You might attribute the word *creativity* to artistic pursuits, but in the way we are using the term, creativity is the ability to conceive something and make it real. Whether you believe it or not, the bottom line is you are the co-creator of your life. You create your home, your family, your income, your personal style, your relationships, your job, your day.

At the root of all that we can see, "Thought is everything," according to Yogananda. He goes on to say, "Thought is the matrix of all creation; thought created everything. If you hold on to that truth with indomitable will, you can materialize any thought."[2] The Yogis teach that creation and nature come from Spirit's thought, and so as Spirit is within us and *is* us as our True Self, so, too, can we create, and we are powerful. And not just little everyday things, but the amazing things you dream of but are scared to sometimes say aloud. The wildly successful business. The beautiful family life. Financial abundance. Real inner peace. Yep, that stuff too.

ARE YOU CREATING AS A BEGGAR OR AS THE TRUE SELF?

Experiencing an awakening and "waking up" out of delusion are common terms associated with enlightenment. We think of sleep as the time when we close our eyes at night and put our heads down on the pillow and drift off. But what if we are sleeping when we think we are awake? Like a kind of sleepwalking where we stumble around in the world and don't know who we really are.

To claim your true power, you must act from your True Self, the part of you that *knows* it is part of Divine intelligence.

When we identify with our small selves, where we experience all the self-doubt and not-enoughness, we disconnect from our True Selves, and we give away our power to create. Think of the analogy of the whole family sitting at the table, where the food gets passed around, and the family members get to eat as much as they want. The beggars sit outside, waiting to be thrown some crumbs here and there. When you identify with your True Self, you are sitting at the table of the feast. There are so many riches that you'll have to turn some of them away. When you identify with your ego, you are identifying with the beggar who will never have enough.

My friend, who we will call Sarah, comes to mind. She is smart and beautiful, owns a business, and is passionate about life, travel, and new experiences. Yet with all her outward success, she longs to have a soul mate to share it with. Since I met her over a decade ago, she hasn't been in a long-term relationship. She is so sure of herself in her business, but in her love life, her self-worth falls to pieces, and she comes from this real lack place versus inner knowing and deserving. She is a beggar when it comes to love.

Yogananda says that any time we begin our prayers by pleading that God help us, we ultimately limit ourselves. Instead, we must first establish the deep belief, the deep *knowing* that the True Self resides inside and is ready to supply us with all that we could ever possibly need. Essentially, you and I and the next person are one with Spirit, with the True Self.

Problems arise, of course, when we don't accept this. As someone who has experienced both ways of living—as a beggar and as a Divine diner—this deep knowing of our intrinsic oneness with Spirit may certainly not come as your first nature. If you've been raised with the idea of God being up there in the sky somewhere, then we have to learn to make this shift. The shift from out there to right inside here.

If you are a child of Source, as the great enlightened ones tell us, it means you acknowledge that you are powerful, that you are a co-creator, and what you create is your Divine birthright. You never have to beg, plead, or grovel. Instead, you can reclaim what we want from that place of knowing you are already part of the kingdom. "No more begging from Him; for you are not a beggar. You are His divine child and inherently have everything He has," Yogananda teaches us.

UNITING WITH SPIRIT FIRST

So what are we supposed to put our energy into? How do we decide what we should create? For Yogananda and just about every spiritual leader, we should seek Spirit first in anything we do. This means putting first things first, and aligning your desires with Spirit's will. That means kicking desire into the backseat while you ride shotgun in the Spirit's SUV of life with the True Self in the driver's seat. By uniting your true identity with the True Self, you access infinite powers to embrace your *true* desires, which are meant to uplift, inspire, and move you toward love, wholeness, and epicness!

Now, I say "true desires" here. What do I mean by this? Well, suppose you desire a new car. When you have this desire, what are you really after? Possibly the freedom that comes with a car you know won't break down. That makes sense. You desire safety. Maybe you want the prestige that comes from a Porsche Cayenne SUV. Well, what you are really desiring (though it may be buried deep inside you) is a feeling of being good enough, important enough, in the eyes of another. Not necessarily a bad thing. But in both instances, they miss the mark in ways because there will always be a pothole that could leave you hanging out on the side of the road. And no matter how many people love you and think you're cool, there will be someone who thinks you're not so cool.

But if you get into alignment and start with Spirit, then everything else falls into place. Then you are looking for safety, not in a steel frame and wheels and not in the arms of adoring fans, but in the consistent love and stability of the True Self.

In other words, put Spirit first and then your desires and the True Self will help you to attain those desires in the most exciting and beneficial way possible. Then it doesn't matter what car you drive—you're not attached to a sports car or a minivan. You know that Spirit will provide your desire with exactly what you need at the right time. We may not be able to attain such lofty acceptance at this time. Still, if we can move closer to detachment from our desires, if we can cultivate an attitude of letting go, we can experience increased Bliss and satisfaction in all that we do.

But does detachment from desire mean that we just become sloths and slugs that don't do anything? Far from it.

Yogananda teaches in his commentary on the ancient Eastern spiritual text the Bhagavad Gita, "Desirelessness does not mean an ambitionless existence. It means to work for the highest and noblest goals without attachment."[3] The way I read Yogananda's position on desire is that it's okay to want things, so long as they don't distract us from our practice and our focus on aligning with the True Self. Only then will all else fall into place. Our desires may naturally shift without our own prodding and pushing and feeling deprived.

CREATING GOOD AND BAD ALIKE

I want to bring up to you in advance that the universe doesn't care about what you set your mind to, good or bad. It doesn't care what you create. If you focus all your attention on the fear of losing a job or doubt your significant other for no reason, then you are on the path to creating what you believe. Once again: you *are* powerful. If you routinely put yourself down, crack jokes about the way you look, constantly reaffirm that you'll never succeed, find love, or have an orgasm, you will get exactly what you focus on. You are the ultimate creator of your own reality, so if you're building a life based on fear or lack, stop it! If your mind is filled with negative crap all the time, negative crap will continue to appear on your doorstep, and you will step in it. And that cosmic crap is no fun to clean off a nice pair of shoes.

Use your powerful creative nature for good. Have faith that things are getting better, that your best is ahead of you, that your greatest love is just on the horizon. This belief isn't wishful thinking; it's putting your faith in your True Self and knowing that the best the world has to offer *will* reveal itself to you when you live from this place of certainty.

The real value of life experiences is not in getting the things we want per se, but in learning that our True Selves are so much more than we think we are. Once we experience our own power for ourselves, we experience this form of enlightenment as truth: we indeed are creators. And we can actually create much larger than we might have thought. In the wise words of Yogananda, "Self-realization is the knowing—in body, mind, and soul—that we are one with the omnipresence of God . . . that we are just as much a part of Him as we ever will be. All we have to do is improve our knowing."[4] Before you can create anything with ease, know this. You are one with the all-powerful Spirit of creation. Now act like it.

CREATING MAGIC

When you connect to your gifts, it is then that you create something beyond extraordinary. Epic stuff. Magical stuff. Stuff that no one else in the entire world can create but you. It is then that we know the truth of when Yogananda says, "You must not let your life run in the ordinary way; do something that nobody else has done, something that will dazzle the world. Show that God's creative principle works in you."[5]

Every one of us has a unique part of us, which others can't replicate. In this way, we are all special. And we don't have to worry about other people "replacing" us, because we can't be exactly replaced. Sure, different people can do the same job or execute the same idea, but only you put your unique spin on it. Have you ever noticed that when two or three people make the exact same recipe, it always tastes different? The chef is always the most essential ingredient in any dish! And it's up to you to tap into your unique specialness. Yogananda counsels us to recognize the tendencies that make each one of us unique.

Creating from your core uniqueness means you are exercising your unique expression of Spirit to help others and yourself grow, which is what we are here to do. It also gives your project or idea the best chance of success because it has your authentic magic in it. When you embody the True Self inside you and create from that place, you create the best stuff possible. From this place, you can be confident of what you are creating. Yet no matter how much of a commercial success it is or not, how big or small by external standards, you have a piece of your heart in your creations, and that's the unique gift you give the world.

You have to first access the higher intelligence inside of you and create from that place. That's where you can pull all the great ideas—from this place of pure potentiality. That's why it's critical to find some space for stillness and silence in your life. Before any big undertaking, meditate first and go within before you attempt to create anything outwardly. Yogananda instructs us, "Before embarking on important undertakings, sit quietly, calm your senses and thoughts, and meditate deeply. You will then be guided by the great creative power of Spirit."[6]

I know many people, and you probably do too, who make lots of money but are miserable. Their hearts are not in what they do. They are restless, dissatisfied, often seeking distractions like after-work drinking every night. Sure, it's great to have money, but if you're reading this book, then you want to create more than just money in your life.

FROM QUANTITATIVE TO QUALITATIVE

It's impossible to put your unique essence into words. Spirit and pure energy, in the true sense, is beyond description. Yet as you channel your unique expression into outer endeavors, words become flesh, relationships begin to blossom, ideas manifest, and you experience a renewal in your ability to create your destiny. We can help ourselves by expanding our vocabulary about what's possible. Here are some examples of adjectives that can start to point to your unique essence:

Warm	Thoughtful	Peaceful
Kind	Compassionate	Open-minded
Loving	Cheerful	Inclusive

You can then start to tap into how your unique essence translates into qualities and how those qualities naturally show up in your world. This then leads to seeing how your gifts can be used in the most effective ways. Here are some examples:

1. You have a particularly warm and comforting way of working with the elderly.

2. You've created a completely different and effective way for helping kids read music.

3. You have a distinctive way of sensing color, making you a spectacular makeup artist on film sets.

4. You have an innate ability to connect deeply with those you physically train and understand how to best motivate and inspire your clients. You decide to parlay it into a whole new type of fitness program and train others under you to take this program to others.

5. You have a natural way of seeing the big picture and breaking it down in a harmonious way with different teams, making you an excellent project manager.

Self-Reflection: Your Energy in Form, Part 1

Please write the answers to these questions in your journal:

1. What are some of the positive traits that others use to describe you?

2. What are some of the ways that you feel that you uniquely do things well? They may seem very small and not so special to you, but note them all, big and so-called tiny.

Don't worry about translating this right now into something bigger; just note these everyday things right now. Here are some examples:

1. I always keep my house super organized.

2. I get along with all my neighbors, even the grumpy ones.

3. When I speak, other people really listen.

4. People come to me for advice about relationships all the time.

5. It's easy for me to understand complicated ideas and break them down to people.

6. I have a green thumb; all my plants thrive.

7. I can create great meals out of whatever I find in the fridge.

We will keep adding on to this exercise in a moment. . . .

LET YOUR HEART LEAD

Passion is a creative tool and a form of intuition. It is the way our bodies and minds know that there is a higher power guiding us to make the right decisions and tap into our talents and willpower. Passion feels like an internal fire and is a clue to where our energies would be most powerful and put to the best and most effective use. It is also linked to inspiration—we take inspired action. And to be inspired is to be full of Spirit.

In psychology, passion is defined as a strong desire for something that people find important. Robert Vallerand, professor of psychology at University of Quebec and expert on motivational processes, and his colleagues propose two types of passion: obsessive and harmonious. Obsessive passion creates control, rigid persistence, and pressure, while harmonious passion is about healthy adaptation and internally feeling drawn to something and then engaging in activities relating to it. We are talking about harmonious passion here, where you feel a natural pull toward something you want to pursue, but without the unhealthy preoccupation that can lead to attachment.

You can't fake passion. You either have it or you don't. It's important to explore your healthy passions, instead of ignoring or suppressing them, to see where they may lead you. Your real passion might be what you're initially drawn to, or what you are currently drawn to might be only part of the path that leads you to your deeper passion and your purpose.

For example, I was very passionate about food at the beginning of my wellness journey. I was bloated and low in energy, full of acne with coarse hair that wouldn't grow. Food, the physical fuel for the body, became a passion that I lived and breathed to learn about every day. When I experienced some tangible physical shifts in my body

after I changed my diet, I pursued studying and researching nutrition almost obsessively, worked at different clin-
ics, and spent hundreds of hours experimenting with
different plant-based recipes.

Yet after writing my first few books that focused on
dietary principles, I could not deny that my passion for
food had expanded. It wasn't that I didn't care about food
anymore, because I still do tremendously. But I had mas-
tered how to eat and had written extensively about it.
After that, I was ready to move on, to keep learning and
growing. I expanded to teaching about a holistic philosophy to feel good that still includes food, but also how to
best care for your body, nourishing your emotional and
mental health, and nurturing your spiritual growth. It's
my 4 Cornerstone Philosophy of True Beauty and Wellness
that I mentioned earlier . . . can you tell how passionate I
am about it?!

All along the way, the goal was and has always been
to help others feel good, but it kept getting deeper and
expanding. As I took steps forward, I could see more than
I could before I took those steps. I began to realize that
while my initial passion for food was important, to really
feel good in the way that I was seeking, I had to go beyond
food. Far beyond. Truly feeling good is about connection—
to others, to our bodies, and specifically and primarily to
the True Self.

What are you passionate about right now? The empha-
sis is on *now*! It might be different from a few years ago or
even a few months ago. As you evolve, it's important to
keep checking in with what is lighting you up, and put
more focus and attention on that passion!

Self-Reflection: Your Energy in Form, Part 2

Please write out in your journal the answers to the following questions:

1. If you are totally open to all possibilities (so don't try to rein yourself in here in any way), what are you really, truly passionate about?

2. How can the positive traits that others naturally notice about me (from Question #1 in Self-Reflection: Your Energy in Form, Part 1) and that I notice about myself support this passion? For example, if you are passionate about starting a mom's advice website, qualities like being warm and inclusive would filter through your writing and draw moms to your site.

3. How can the unique ways I do things well (from Question #2 in Self-Reflection: Your Energy in Form, Part 1), even the things that are unrelated, somehow translate or be part of my passions? For example, suppose you are able to get along with all your neighbors, even the grumpy ones. In that case, you will be able to peacefully moderate the chat groups within your mom's website, helping to smooth over arguments between members, for instance, and ensure everyone feels welcome.

4. What are some of the ways I can translate my passions into creations in the world? What am I meant to create right now? Be sure to do your meditation before you answer. It can be a shorter one, but please close your eyes, go into your meditation posture, and meditate. If you can't do this right now, then wait until after your next morning or evening meditation and journal the answers to these questions.

EXPAND THE CIRCLE

When you expand your ideas to include the welfare of others, your ability to manifest explodes. Why is that? Because we move from isolation and separation to becoming and serving the whole. And when we are part of the whole, then we have the whole access to our God-given powers flowing through us. Think of it like blood flowing in our bodies. When blood moves freely, it provides its life-giving powers to all parts of us, our organs, muscles, and brain. But if blood clots in dangerous ways—if it stops flowing freely and collects and builds up in certain areas, what can happen? Stroke, heart attack, death. The same can happen to us spiritually if we are not flowing.

It's fantastic to love your family and your closest inner circle so much, but we must expand that love out into the world. This is key, because it goes back to our recurring theme of enlightenment: expansion. Anytime you act in a limited and small way, you cut off your potential—your potential for growth, abundance, love, everything. This means the more you give, the more you get back. While this might sound cliché, it is true nonetheless.

Being united with all our brothers and sisters is our natural state. We aren't meant to live separate lives where we think only of ourselves. There is a real lack mentality when we do that, and it cuts us off from the universal supply of abundance. So, know that if you want to supercharge your life, be sure to include the good of all in the things you do, say, and think.

Brian Tracy, an author who has written over 80 books on success and personal growth, explains it best when he says, "Successful people are always looking for opportunities to help others. Unsuccessful people are always asking, 'What's in it for me?'"[7]

This brings to mind Scott Harrison, who I loved interviewing for my podcast. Scott was a big party dude who flew around the world as a club promoter. Despite all the material success in the "bottles and models" departments, as he described to me on the show, he started feeling emptier and emptier. Life became shallow, and all the excitement that he loved so much dissipated into nothing.

Long story short, Scott began to realize that he had spent a lot of time focusing on himself and little time focusing on others. He soon started volunteering and began to find a new sense of what it meant to be truly alive. In time, he turned his attention toward helping others full time, and he used his marketing skills to found Charity: Water. This nonprofit organization raises millions of dollars every year to build wells for thousands of people in communities that previously had no access to fresh water. Aligning with the greater good was key to his success.

Try it for yourself and notice how much the law of supply will expand when you intentionally use your will to help benefit the greater good, in whatever ways speak to you from your heart. And know that as Yogananda teaches, "As soon as you love not only your family, but give that love to all, you are going toward God."[8]

DYNAMIC WILLPOWER

Once you have your idea or ideas built around your passion, it's time to use your will and power to act. The will is paramount in Yogananda's teaching. We also discussed will in Chapter 12, but it is really important to understand how it relates to creating what you want, so we are now going to discuss it further and with more detail.

When we talk about willpower, we are essentially talking about making things happen, whether it's running a race, making dinner, saving money, raising a child, and so on. According to the general consensus of psychologists, part of the definition of willpower is the ability to delay gratification, resisting short-term temptations to meet long-term goals.[9]

Yogananda often used the term *dynamic will power* to refer to using your will in stronger and stronger ways, no matter what the circumstances. "Carrying a thought with dynamic will power means holding to it until that thought pattern develops dynamic force. When a thought is made dynamic by will force, it can create or rearrange the atoms into the desired pattern according to the mental blueprint you have created," Yogananda teaches.[10]

Thought *is* powerful. More powerful than you may realize. When Yogananda was referring to the "mental blueprint" above, he was referring to creating from your thoughts. Something that backs this up in science is the discovery of "mirror neurons." According to Dr. Srini Pillay, a Harvard-trained physician, when we observe someone doing something, the same pattern of brain activation allows that observer to set up a simulation as if they are doing the same thing.[11] These activations in the brain are seen in the premotor and parietal cortex of the brain. So we can theorize that if you can observe your goals and dreams in your mind, your brain can start to create neural patterns as if those things are already happening and help make them into reality.

You cling to the inner knowing of your True Self, and you see it through to completion. If you keep believing and working toward your goal, Divine power will come in to support your efforts. We aren't meant to drift along and just declare what we want and then sit back and wait for someone to hand it to us. We are to use our God-given will.

Details can always be figured out, so don't worry about that part right now. Lead with your initiative to come up with new, creative ideas. It's inside of you.

Some psychological researchers have theorized that willpower is finite and connected only to a limited reserve of mental energy. Once you run out of that energy, well, there goes your willpower and also your self-control.[12] However, in recent studies, this has been challenged. This includes research from Stanford psychologist Carol Dweck and her colleagues, published in *Proceedings of the National Academy of Sciences*. Dweck concluded that signs of running low on willpower and self-control were observed only in test subjects who *believed* willpower was a limited resource. Those participants who did not see willpower as finite did not show such signs.[13]

Michael Inzlicht, a psychology professor at the University of Toronto and the principal investigator at the Toronto Laboratory for Social Neuroscience, also believes willpower is not a finite resource but instead acts similarly to an emotion. He theorizes that your willpower can ebb and flow based on what's happening to you and how you feel, and you can't run out of it, just as you can't run out of emotions like anger and joy.[14]

Some will say that you can't just rely on your willpower in your everyday life and tasks, let's say, for improving your personal fitness. Sometimes we think it has to be more complicated than that, and we need other tools. Maybe, you reason, to get into shape, you have to mix in all different kinds of workouts, seek out more or different equipment, use online apps to keep you motivated, and make space in your schedule for working out.

Now, I'm not criticizing these ideas. All of those means may be totally useful and part of creating the goal, but it all starts with your will if you want to increase your fitness. You still have to think of getting in shape first and then commit to the idea with your dynamic will. You don't let Netflix sidetrack you from getting a good night's sleep. Once you commit, you follow it through until you are truly fit!

Yogananda not only taught that we have this powerful Divine will, but that we are *supposed* to use it. Yogananda says, "Remember, God is with you. You are exercising His power, which you have borrowed from Him, and when you do that He will be nearer to you to help you."[15] Yogananda's guru, Swami Sri Yukteswar, said that whatever you imagine will be created for you if your will is strong. Could it really be that simple?

Well, yes, but simple does not mean easy. It means using the gift of your will and channeling it into hard work. Yogananda says, "A home will not be dropped down to you from heaven; you will have to pour forth will power continuously through constructive actions. . . . Even if there is nothing in the world to conform to your wish, when your will persists, the desired result will somehow manifest."

Tap into your will, and you will create magic. You *are* a creator by nature, so bring forth the creations into the world that no one else can bring forth but you.

Practical Tips for Being a Creator

1. **Meditate to align yourself with your best ideas.** One of the best times to ask for guidance is after doing your meditation practice, when your mind is still and you have connected with your True Self. If you connect inward first, you will be able to bypass the mind's logic and get down to deeper intuition, where the highest and best ideas are available to you.

   Yogananda stressed the importance of always contacting Spirit first before any decisions or important endeavors. Sit quietly, calm your breath and thoughts, and let your senses calm down. Practice the basic meditation techniques in this book and meditate as deeply as you can. Then you will be guided by what Yogananda calls "the great creative power of Spirit."

2. **Find times for silence.** When we talk all the time, we find that our creative energy is always flowing out, and we don't have any space for listening, including to our intuition and guidance, on moving forward when we're working on manifesting something. Yogananda says that in times of stillness and introspection, we move away from "frantic reasonings" and instead go toward a "stilling of thoughts, which are then replaced with intuitive perception."[16] My daily one-hour walk is my precious silent time. I commit to carving out time for it, because it's true that when I am home that silent time might soon be overrun by one of the

kids or a team member or hubby coming to me for something!

3. **Use visualization.** Visualize the end result of your creative idea, even if you don't yet have all the answers or all the steps on how to get there. Imagine and feel the excitement around the details of your end idea as clearly as possible. Be sure to include the visions of how others would benefit, how the quality of their lives would somehow improve.

4. **Conviction.** Visualization alone isn't going to get you there. Next, you have to use the strength of your willpower to turn your visualization— that which you want to create—into a clear conviction. And "when you can hold that conviction against all odds," Yogananda says, "it will come true."[17]

5. **Write it down.** When you are first starting to germinate the very beginning of an idea, and all the way through the process, be sure to write down your ideas in your journal. It's the first step in transmuting your idea or vision into reality. Try writing in your own hand rather than typing, as research shows that writing by hand can actually engage your brain far more.[18]

6. **Be the manager of your own habits.** Yogananda spoke at length about the enormous impact our habits have on our lives, including on our ability to create our dreams into success. He says, "Why is it that you sometimes find yourself acting, or reacting, contrary to your real desires? Because over a period of time you have built up

habits that are contrary to those desires, and your actions automatically flatter your habits. You must first establish habits that will influence your actions to cater to your true ideals."[19]

Ask yourself if your daily habits are supporting or detracting from what you want to create. If you want to create optimal health, but you still haven't kicked your daily cigarette habit, you might want to step back and rethink. Or if you want to create a successful business, but you continually sleep past your morning staff meetings, you're not reinforcing that with your actions. So watch all your daily habits and commit to improving or dropping them as you see fit.

7. **Manage other people well.** Along the journey of creating your dreams, whether that's a healthy family life, or launching a new jewelry line or wreath business on Etsy, we need to enlist other people in countless other ways. This includes manufacturers, customers, family, friends, your kids' teachers and coaches, a sales team, a web team, and so on! So managing other people well is super important. Human relations can be dicey on all fronts, because everyone has their own sensitivities and triggers, including those you work with, so it's important to handle everyone in the best possible way. Yogananda tells us, "If you approach others not with the attitude of bossing or anger but with sincere love, there are very few people who will misunderstand you."[20]

Try to let your heart lead instead of the ego, and keep the greater good, win-win picture in mind in communication and decision-making to support your successful creations.

8. **Keep the doubters in the dark.** When your dreams are just starting off, as the tiniest of little seed babies, you might want to nurture them quietly and privately for a time. Even well-meaning loved ones can cast doubt on your burgeoning willpower with their words, or even their looks of disapproval. Give your little seeds of new intentions some breathing room to take root before sharing them with others, to maintain your utmost focus. You don't want to spend energy convincing others of the viability of your goal when you can use that energy to work on the goal itself.

9. **Persistence.** Using your will is like training for a marathon or a mountain-climbing expedition. One day you might run like a champ. Another day you might struggle to do half of what you did earlier in the week. Never give up. Stay focused on your goal and know that you hold your creation in your hands. As Yogananda says, "As soon as your attention is focused, the Power of all powers will come, and with that you can achieve spiritual, mental, and material success."[21]

Chapter 20

PRACTICE:
Meditation, PART III:
EXPANDING THE LIGHT

*"The devotee is aware that the most important
objective in life is to attain the goal of Self-realization:
to know through meditation his true soul nature
and its oneness with ever blissful Spirit."*

— PARAMAHANSA YOGANANDA[1]

You might hear the phrase "love and light" tossed
around. We've covered love, and we've discussed light in
some instances, but what *is* the light part exactly? Light is
beyond any form. Light is pure energy. Cosmic Energy or
Cosmic Light is referred to in the Gita as *Vivasvat*: "one who
shines forth or diffuses light." Yogananda explains, "This
omnipresent Cosmic Energy or Light exists in man as the
microcosmic sun of the spiritual eye, which becomes vis-
ible during meditation when the devotee's consciousness
and the dual current of the two physical eyes is concentrated at the point between the eyebrows."[2]

We can access the light within all of us by focusing on our third eye, as we discussed in the Chapter 10, Practice: Meditation, Part II: The Third Eye. The light comes into our being through the medulla and then radiates to the third eye, which allows us to see with God's eyes. In our quest to really know the True Self and access the light, it is essential to spend more time in deeper and deeper focus on the third eye in meditation. When we put our full focus on this specific spot, we start to align with the energy there. We can then begin to know our true nature. First, it may start as a mental idea: "Oh yeah, my third eye is where I'm supposed to focus when I meditate!" Then it transitions into an actual experience, a feeling of merging, where you feel Spirit as every cell of your body. As you persist in your practice of meditation, over time you will begin to experience the light of the spiritual eye. Yogananda says, "The upwardly climbing yogi experiences the inner light first, then cosmic perception."[3]

And as you continue to expand, you will also see Spirit reflected back to you in all things—people, pets, the birds outside your window, the room around you, your furniture, plants, the trees, the buildings, the villages, the cities, everywhere and in everything. There is nothing that exists outside of Source. There is nothing that wasn't created by Source. That means that everything around you contains within it the Divine. The more you meditate, the more you'll begin to see this. In fact, the word *rishi*, which refers to India's wise spiritual people, literally translates as "seer." Rishis are the ones who have seen with their third eye and live on earth from that place of much greater expanded awareness. They literally see more truth. And guess what? You and I can work to see more too. It's a path that's free and open to all of us, not just a few privileged holy people.

The first time I felt an experience of embodied awareness of light, I was on a walk by myself in the mountains around my home. I looked up at the sunlight flooding through some oak trees, and in one instance I felt a full flash of knowingness. It was a magical, life-changing experience. I could feel light in every cell. It was like a huge searchlight with a million watts of power beamed down and then through every millimeter of me. I felt a sense of purification and focus. All my insecurities, fears, and worries dissolved. All the little daily stuff, the annoyances, the sense of lack, feelings of not being enough, felt completely ridiculous and irrelevant.

That experience lasted only a few minutes, but it did change me. These experiences now come more regularly to me in meditation, and more often now, like that experience, they show up spontaneously in my daily life. This meditation practice can give you a peek at the overwhelming levels of the love of Spirit. This love trumps any love we've felt here in this world, yet it allows you to open your heart more and trust and love yourself and others more unconditionally.

Now the truth is, you already have a level of these kinds of experiences in your life. You just might not notice them or realize they are happening. You could be driving in your car, changing your baby's diaper, folding laundry, making a smoothie, kissing your beloved, or just walking to get the mail, and you have a flash of "knowing," a moment when everything feels good, feels right, feels centered. When this happens, you are having a True Self sighting! You might not feel joyful, but you're not feeling sad either. You just are, present in the moment. Oftentimes when we notice these moments, we fall out of them. And that's okay. What meditation does is help you experience more of these "knowing" moments for longer and longer periods and go deeper into them and into feelings of complete unity with all.

To know the True Self is through experience. All the wisdom we've been discussing throughout the book is essential to deeper understanding and getting your mind out of the way. But ultimately, it's all paving the path for effective meditation, the true way to experience Spirit.

ONENESS

This meditation practice focuses on expansion. It is based on a beginning technique that Yogananda taught to show us that when we expand our consciousness, we go beyond the little ego, the little self, and realize the truth of Oneness.

When we get Oneness, it is a massive game-changer! Oneness converts our perspective from smallness and competition into merging and harmony. The great creative power manifests in infinite ways, through all of us and all things. That's what Oneness really means. While we may look and act differently and have different bodies and different forms, we are all of the same source. Therefore we are all connected, and we can also tap into all things. It's so powerful. Talk about being more than you think you are! Yogananda says, "All mankind are not only our friends, but our Self! Friends are God in disguise."[4]

Let's get into our practice now. Let's get going and journey into the Light.

1. **Get into the proper position in your meditation seat.** Be sure to lift your spine.

2. **Start with an intention.** Focus your mind, and dedicate your practice.

3. **Do the preliminary breathing exercise by Paramahansa Yogananda of tensing and relaxing your body (described in detail in Chapter 7).**[5] Here are some key reminders of this technique:

   As you inhale, and holding in the breath, tense the whole body to a count of six. Next, expel the breath in a double exhale of "huh, huhhh," a sound made by the breath rushing out. Relax all the tension in your body at the same time. Repeat this exercise three times.

4. **Breathe and do the Expanding the Gaps Practice.** Ideally this would be at least 5–10 or more minutes, as you are getting started with your overall practice (more detail back in Chapter 4).

5. **See the light.** After going through the initial steps to ground yourself in your meditation, lift your internal gaze to your third eye. Start repeating the simple mantra (Peace or *Shanti* or another word you resonate with) and begin visualizing a white light. Imagine the point of light is centered right in your third eye. You can even lightly touch your finger to that spot (between your eyebrows and about half of an inch higher) to help you home in on that specific spot.

Be sure to do this part of the practice for at least 2–3 minutes when starting out, and for longer as you get more into your practice.

6. **Expand the light across your entire body.** Now imagine the light starts expanding into a bigger and bigger circle of light, until it encompasses your entire forehead. Keep expanding the light across your face and allow it to spread down your neck and shoulders, into your arms, your torso, and down into your legs. Imagine the light fully saturating every cell of your body. Stay in that pulsating light for a few moments at least, or for as long as it feels good to you, until you feel complete with the exercise.

7. **Expand the light beyond your body.** Now imagine the light expanding and growing beyond your body, in 360 degrees, all around you, as if your body were a giant disco ball radiating light in all directions. See and feel the light shining into the chair or the space around you, into the room and the house or building you are in. Witness it as it expands into the land all around.

Keep envisioning this light as it grows beyond what you can see, beyond your town, village, or city, your state, the country you live in.

Keep going! Visualize the light going beyond the oceans, over the mountains, to all countries and across the planet, until the entire world is lit up with this brilliant white light. Then go even beyond the planet and see the light filling the cosmos—the stars and other planets and the black spaces in between the entire multiverse.

Stay in this space of expanded awareness for a few minutes.

8. **Integrate the feelings of Oneness.** As you feel the light that started as a single point expand to include the entire universe and beyond, remind yourself that you are part of all things, and connected to all things. And there is nothing and nobody that is outside of the light, outside of you, really.

This is something that can't really be put into words. It's an experience that will deepen over time, as you go about your practice, experiencing no real hard boundaries of anything. Nothing is really "separate" from you. Don't believe me? Try this little thought experiment.

Imagine that you are standing three feet away from a friend or loved one. Picture in your mind a flying camera hovering in the middle of the space between you and your friend. Then, using a remote control with a video screen on it, you send the camera up to the sky 500 feet, then 1,000 feet, then a mile, then 10 miles. What do you see? As the camera rises into the sky, you see that the distance between you and your friend becomes smaller and smaller. At a certain point you'll see that you actually share the same space. And as you send the camera traveling into outer space, you see that you share the same space with everyone in the world. That is the glory of the True Self: it sees up close and it sees from a distance. It sees the awesome differences that make you, you, and me, me, but it also sees that we are really all part of one creation.

It might take some time to integrate Oneness beyond an intellectual concept to a true knowingness. But you can start visualizing it and becoming open to it.

Oneness can only come after you can see the light in yourself first. So be patient! Keep going with your practice. It took me some time to see the light inside of me and then outwardly, but it did come. And it will come to you too. The exponential lightness you will feel, the deeper love and peace inside of you, is worth everything.

9. **Close in gratitude.** As always, we want to express our gratitude for being alive. It is a true gift to even be on this path in the first place.

When you've completed your practice, bring your hands together in Anjali mudra, or prayer position, in front of your heart. As we always close our meditations, take a moment to be grateful for Spirit, your breath, these teachings, your practice, and whatever else spontaneously arises from your heart. You can also pray, if that resonates with you.

Chapter 21

YOU ARE THE TRUE SELF

*"When you go beyond the consciousness
of this world, knowing that you are not the body
or the mind, and yet aware as never before that you
exist—that divine consciousness is what you are. You are
That in which is rooted everything in the universe."*

— PARAMAHANSA YOGANANDA[1]

Dear Reader,

Imagine you are sitting on a beautiful beach. The ocean waves are crashing before you. You feel the warm, nourishing sunlight on your skin, and your feet sink into the beautiful earth as the cool sand and water swirl around your ankles. Relaxing into this experience, you are overcome by peace. You are truly blissed out!

Then out of nowhere, your thoughts start to churn. You begin to feel anxious and worried. "Did I leave on the stove? Did that check cash? Oh no, I forgot to e-mail my co-worker. I hope my friend's doctor appointment goes well. What if it doesn't?"

What was once a feeling of peace has turned to anxiety. Your body tightens and you feel the familiar tension building in your neck. Your breathing becomes shallow, and you wonder why you are on the beach in the first place instead of off getting more work done back at home.

Just at that moment you feel a hand on your shoulder. It feels like the most comforting, nurturing touch, and you feel a surge of calm flow through your whole being. You are instantly back to a peaceful state, except now you feel even more peaceful than when you first walked onto the beach. You *know—you really know*—how supported you truly are. And you realize that, while everything might not be right in the world, you feel prepared and confident to deal with each moment as it comes.

That hand on your shoulder is the True Self. The True Self that is always traveling with you in each and every moment, like your portable best friend that isn't even next to you or even in your pocket—she is within you. *She is you!* The time for seeking answers outside of yourself is over. The restless searching for joy and peace, it turns out, was never for anything in the external world. That energy you felt—those butterflies in the stomach, that desire to move your body, to go places, to experience new things, that flutter in your hands—was just the True Self trying to get your attention.

All of these beautiful, powerful, Divine qualities that we discussed throughout this book radiate out of the True Self. They are limbs and organs of the body of the True Self that work together to make you, you. All you have to do is tune in to these parts of your True Self, pay attention to them, honor them, and let them do their job, and you can live the life of your dreams.

While writing this book, I wrote this affirmation in my journal, and I keep coming back to it:

The more I identify with the light inside of me,
The brighter I become.

Let your light, dear reader, radiate with the intensity, the vibrancy, the strength of the sun and moon! This is how we become enlightened, by letting the light inside of us shine brightly day and night.

It has been a great honor for me to be with you on this path, and to share the teachings of the great yoga guru Paramahansa Yogananda. My deepest intention with this book is to lead you to the peace and joy that is already inside of you and to offer some tools to help you build a life of loving awareness. I hope when you look in the mirror that you see a new you, the real you, that may have been hiding in your life.

Like my mom said to me years ago, you are more than you think you are.

So much more.

Go forth and be *you*.

With great love, your friend on the path,

Kimberly

RESOURCES

Please find more information on Paramahansa Yogananda and Kriya Yoga at https://yogananda.org

The Self-Realization Fellowship Lessons can be found at https://yogananda.org/lessons-programs

Join the Solluna Circle at www.mysolluna.com or in the Solluna by Kimberly Snyder free app (in the membership section).

Recommended Reading

Autobiography of a Yogi, by Paramahansa Yogananda

Other books by Paramahansa Yogananda:

Metaphysical Meditations

The Yoga of the Gita

Inner Peace

To Be Victorious in Life

Where There Is Light

Transcending the Levels of Consciousness, by David Hawkins, MD, PhD

Letting Go, by David Hawkins, MD, PhD

Radical Beauty, co-authored by Deepak Chopra and Kimberly Snyder

Micro-shifts, by Gary Jansen

ENDNOTES

Chapter 1

1. Paramahansa Yogananda, "Illumine Your Life with the Flame of Self-Realization," *Self-Realization*, Winter 2011.
2. Paramahansa Yogananda, "How to Use Thoughts of Immortality to Awaken Your True Self," *Self-Realization*, Winter 2005.
3. Paramahansa Yogananda, *Highest Achievements Through Self-Realization* (Los Angeles: Self-Realization Fellowship, 2019) flipbook.

Chapter 2

1. Paramahansa Yogananda, *The Divine Romance: Collected Talks and Essays on Realizing God in Daily Life, Volume II* (Los Angeles: Self-Realization Fellowship, 1986).
2. Bert Tuk, "Overstimulation of the Inhibitory Nervous System Plays a Role in the Pathogenesis of Neuromuscular and Neurological Diseases: a Novel Hypothesis" [Version 2; peer review: 2 approved], *F1000Res.* 5: 1435 (August 19, 2016). doi: 10.12688/f1000research.8774.1.
3. "Shadow (Psychology)," Wikipedia, modified April 26, 2021, https://en.wikipedia.org/wiki/Shadow_(psychology).
4. Ibid.

Chapter 3

1. Paramahansa Yogananda, *Sayings of Paramahansa Yogananda* (Los Angeles: Self-Realization Fellowship, 1980), 95.
2. Paramahansa Yogananda, *God Talks with Arjuna: the Bhagavad Gita* (Los Angeles: Self-Realization Fellowship, 1995).
3. Paramahansa Yogananda, *The Divine Romance: Collected Talks and Essays on Realizing God in Daily Life, Volume II* (Los Angeles: Self-Realization Fellowship, 1986), 93.
4. Ibid., 94.
5. Ibid., 93.

Chapter 4

1. Paramahansa Yogananda, *Lesson 4: Self-Realization Fellowship Lessons* (Los Angeles: Self-Realization Fellowship, 2019).

2. Braboszcz, et al., "Increased Gamma Brainwave Amplitude Compared to Control in Three Different Meditation Traditions," *PLoS One* 12(1): e0170647 (January 24, 2017). doi:10.1371/journal.pone.0170647.

3. Jennifer Larson, "What to Know About Gamma Brain Waves," *Healthline*, June 22, 2020, https://www.healthline.com/health/gamma-brain-waves.

4. Tang, et al., "Induced Gamma Activity in EEG Represents Cognitive Control During Detecting Emotional Expressions," *Annu Int Conf IEEE Eng Med Biol Soc.* (2011): 1717–20. doi: 10.1109/IEMBS.2011.6090492.

5. Ibid.

6. Russo, M. A., Santarelli, D. M., and O'Rourke, D., "The Physiological Effects of Slow Breathing in the Healthy Human," *Breathe (Sheff)* 13(4) (2017): 298–309. doi:10.1183/20734735.009817.

7. Michael J. Aminoff, *Encyclopedia of the Neurological Sciences* (Elsevier Science Inc., 2003), 54.

Chapter 5

1. Paramahansa Yogananda, *Where There Is Light: Insight and Inspiration for Meeting Life's Challenges* (Los Angeles: Self-Realization Fellowship, 2015), 189.

2. Paramahansa Yogananda, *The Divine Romance: Collected Talks and Essays on Realizing God in Daily Life, Volume II* (Los Angeles: Self-Realization Fellowship, 2017), 11.

3. Ibid., 14.

4. Ibid., 15.

5. Ibid., 5.

6. Ibid., 5.

7. Mark Horoszowski, "5 Surprising Benefits of Volunteering," *Forbes*, March 19, 2015, https://www.forbes.com/sites/nextavenue/2015/03/19/5-surprising-benefits-of-volunteering/?sh=2d7db5b6127b.

8. Paramahansa Yogananda, *Journey to Self-Realization: Collected Talks and Essays on Realizing God in Daily Life, Volume III* (Los Angeles: Self-Realization Fellowship, 1997), 385.

9. Ibid., 160.

10. Witvliet, C.V.O., Ludwig, T. E., and Vander Laan, K. L., "Granting Forgiveness of Harboring Grudges: Implications for Emotion, Physiology, and Health," *Psychological Science* 12 (2001): 117–123.

11. At the Biocybernaut Institute in Sedona, Arizona.

12. "Giving Thanks Can Make You Happier," Harvard Health Publishing, August 14, 2021, https://www.health.harvard.edu/healthbeat/giving-thanks-can-make-you-happier.

13. Paramahansa Yogananda, *The Divine Romance: Collected Talks and Essays on Realizing God in Daily Life Volume II* (Los Angeles: Self-Realization Fellowship, 2017).

Chapter 6

1. Paramahansa Yogananda, *Sayings of Paramahansa Yogananda* (Los Angeles: Self-Realization Fellowship, 1980).

2. Wayne Dyer, *The Power of Awakening* (Carlsbad, California: Hay House, 2020), 1.

3. Paramahansa Yogananda, *God Talks with Arjuna: The Bhagavad Gita* (Los Angeles: Self-Realization Fellowship, 1995), 440.

4. Paramahansa Yogananda, *The Divine Romance: Collected Talks and Essays on Realizing God in Daily Life* (Los Angeles: Self-Realization Fellowship, 2011), 144.

5. Ibid., 147.

6. Dan Zahavi, *Self and Other: Exploring Subjectivity, Empathy and Shame* (Oxford: Oxford University Press, 2014).

7. "Shame and Guilt: The Good, the Bad, and the Ugly," YouTube video, 1:12:15, "ResearchChannel," February 9, 2008, https://youtu.be/febgutDYP7w.

8. Fergus, et al., "Shame- and Guilt-Proneness: Relationships with Anxiety Disorder Symptoms in a Clinical Sample," *Journal of Anxiety Disorders* 24, no. 8 (June 11, 2010): 811–5. doi: 10.1016/j.janxdis.2010.06.002.

9. Lewis, M. and Ramsay, D., "Cortisol Response to Embarrassment and Shame," *Child Dev 73* (2002): 1034–45. doi: 10.1111/1467-8624.00455.

10. Dickerson, S. S., et al., "Immunological Effects of Induced Shame and Guilt," *Psychosomatic Medicine* 6 (2004): 124–31.

11. Paramahansa Yogananda, *Autobiography of a Yogi* (Los Angeles: The Self-Realization Fellowship, 1946).

12. Paramahansa Yogananda, *The Divine Romance: Collected Talks and Essays on Realizing God in Daily Life*, Volume II (Los Angeles: Self-Realization Fellowship, 2011).

Chapter 7

1. Paramahansa Yogananda, *God Talks with Arjuna: The Bhagavad Gita* (Los Angeles: Self-Realization Fellowship, 1995).
2. Yogananda, Paramahansa. *Where There Is Light: Insight and Inspiration for Meeting Life's Challenges.* (Los Angeles: Self-Realization Fellowship, 1989).

Chapter 8

1. Paramahansa Yogananda, *Journey to Self-Realization: Collected Talks and Essays on Realizing God in Daily Life, Volume III* (Los Angeles: Self-Realization Fellowship, 1997).
2. Yaribeygi, H., et al., "The Impact of Stress on Body Function: A Review," *EXCLI Journal* 16 (July 21, 2017):1057–1072. doi:10.17179/excli2017-480.
3. Melchior, M., et al., "Work Stress Precipitates Depression and Anxiety in Young, Working Women and Men," *Psychological Medicine* 37, no. 8 (2007):1119–1129. doi:10.1017/S0033291707000414.
4. HeartMath, "How Stress Affects the Body," *Health & Wellness* (blog), December 6, 2017, https://www.heartmath.com/blog/health-and-wellness/how-stress-affects-the-body/.
5. Paramahansa Yogananda, *Where There Is Light: Insight and Inspiration for Meeting Life's Challenges* (Los Angeles: Self-Realization Fellowship, 1989).
6. Paramahansa Yogananda, *Journey to Self-Realization: Collected Talks and Essays on Realizing God in Daily Life*, Volume III (Los Angeles: Self-Realization Fellowship, 1997).

Chapter 9

1. Yogananda, Paramahansa, *Journey to Self-Realization: Collected Talks and Essays on Realizing God in Daily Life, Volume III* (Los Angeles: Self-Realization Fellowship, 1997), 219.
2. Ibid.
3. Ibid.
4. Ibid., 295.
5. Paramahansa Yogananda, "Self-Realization: Knowing Your Infinite Nature," *Self-Realization*, Fall 2003.

Chapter 10

1. Paramahansa Yogananda, *Where There Is Light: Insight and Inspiration for Meeting Life's Challenges* (Los Angeles: Self-Realization Fellowship, 2015), 25.
2. Ibid., 23.

Chapter 11

1. Paramahansa Yogananda, *Autobiography of a Yogi* (Los Angeles: Self-Realization Fellowship, 1946).
2. Ibid., 112.
3. Lufityanto, G., Donkin, C., and Pearson, J. "Measuring Intuition: Nonconscious Emotional Information Boosts Decision Accuracy and Confidence," *Psychological Science* (April 6, 2016). doi: 10.1177/0956797616629403.
4. Gigerenzer, G., and Gaissmaier, W., "Heuristic Decision Making," *Annual Review of Psychology* 62 (January 2011) 451–482.
5. Dijksterhuis, et al., "On Making the Right Choice: The Deliberation-Without-Attention Effect," *Science* 311 (February 17, 2006): 1005–1007.
6. Matthew Hutson, "8 Truths About Intuition: What to Know About What You Don't Know," *Psychology Today*, December 19, 2019, https://www.psychologytoday.com/us/articles/201912/8-truths-about-intuition.
7. Ibid., 302.
8. Paramahansa Yogananda, *The Divine Romance: Collected Talks and Essays on Realizing God in Daily Life, Volume II* (Los Angeles: Self-Realization Fellowship, 1986).
9. Ibid.
10. Paramahansa Yogananda, *Journey to Self-Realization: Collected Talks and Essays on Realizing God in Daily Life, Volume III* (Los Angeles: Self-Realization Fellowship, 1997), 111.
11. Ibid., 309.
12. Ibid., 10.
13. Ibid., 73.
14. Ibid., 204.

Chapter 12

1. Paramahansa Yogananda, *The Divine Romance: Collected Talks and Essays on Realizing God in Daily Life*, Volume II (Los Angeles: Self-Realization Fellowship, 1986).
2. Lo'eau LaBonta, "Human Energy Converted to Electricity," Stanford University, December 6, 2014, http://large.stanford.edu/courses/2014/ph240/labonta1/#:~:text=The%20average%20human%2C%20at%20rest,can%20output%20over%202%2C000%20watts.
3. Harinath, et al., "Effects of Hatha Yoga and Omkar Meditation on Cardiorespiratory Performance, Psychologic Profile, and Melatonin Secretion," *Journal of Alternative and Complementary Medicine* 10, no. 2 (April 2004): 261–8.

4. Lucas, et al., "A Prospective Association Between Hypotension and Idiopathic Chronic Fatigue," *Journal of Hypertension* 22, no. 4 (April 2004): 691–695.

5. Stephanie Willerth, *Engineering Neural Tissue from Stem Cells* (London: Academic Press, 2017), PDF, iv.

6. Deligkaris, et al., "Job Burnout and Cognitive Functioning: A Systematic Review," *Work & Stress*, 28, no. 2 (2014): 107–123. doi: 10.1080/02678373.2014.909545.

7. David Hawkins, *Letting Go: The Pathway of Surrender* (Carlsbad, California: Hay House, 2012), 11.

8. Ibid., 11.

9. Ibid., 20.

10. Paramahansa Yogananda, *The Divine Romance: Collected Talks and Essays on Realizing God in Daily Life,* Volume II (Los Angeles: Self-Realization Fellowship, 1986).

Chapter 13

1. Paramahansa Yogananda, "Energization," *Self-Realization,* Summer 2016.

2. Sandra Anderson, "The 5 Prana Vayus Chart," Yoga International, https://yogainternational.com/article/view/the-5-prana-vayus-chart.

3. Paramahansa Yogananda, "The Divine Art of Erasing Age and Creating Vitality," *Self-Realization,* Fall 2007.

Chapter 14

1. Paramahansa Yogananda, *The Divine Romance: Collected Talks and Essays on Realizing God in Daily Life, Volume II* (Los Angeles: Self-Realization Fellowship, 1986), 330.

2. Ibid.

3. Paramahansa Yogananda, *Autobiography of a Yogi* (Los Angeles: Self-Realization Fellowhip, 1946).

4. Paramahansa Yogananda, *The Divine Romance: Collected Talks and Essays on Realizing God in Daily Life, Volume II* (Los Angeles: Self-Realization Fellowship, 1986), 330.

Chapter 15

1. Paramahansa Yogananda, *The Divine Romance: Collected Talks and Essays on Realizing God in Daily Life, Volume II* (Los Angeles: Self-Realization Fellowship, 1986), 330.

2. Paramahansa Yogananda, *Para-Grams* (Los Angeles: Self-Realization Fellowship).

3. Paramahansa Yogananda, *Where There Is Light: Insight and Inspiration for Meeting Life's Challenges* (Los Angeles: Self Realization Fellowship, 2015), 87.

4. Hunt, T., and Schooler, J., "The 'Easy Part' of the Hard Problem: A Resonance Theory of Consciousness," *Authorea* (January 04, 2019). doi: 10.22541/au.154659223.37007989.

5. Ibid.

6. Steven Strogatz, *Sync: How Order Emerges from Chaos in the Universe, Nature and Daily Life* (New York: Hyperion, 2003).

7. Ibid., 11.

8. Rollin McCraty, *Science of the Heart, Volume 2: Exploring the Role of the Heart in Human Performance* (Boulder Creek, California: HeartMath, 2015), 1.

9. David Hawkins, *Power Vs. Force: The Hidden Determinants of Human Behavior* (Carlsbad, California: Hay House, 2012), 55.

10. Ibid., 26.

11. Ibid., 26.

12. Paramahansa Yogananda, *Autobiography of a Yogi* (Los Angeles: Self-Realization Fellowship, 1946).

Chapter 16

1. Paramahansa Yogananda, *Scientific Healing Affirmations* (Los Angeles: Self-Realization Fellowship, 1929).

2. Ibid.

3. Ibid.

4. Paramahansa Yogananda, *Where There Is Light: Insight and Inspiration for Meeting Life's Challenges* (Los Angeles: Self Realization Fellowship, 2015), 42.

5. Paramahansa Yogananda, *Scientific Healing Affirmations* (Los Angeles: Self-Realization Fellowship, 1929).

Chapter 17

1. Paramahansa Yogananda, *Journey to Self-Realization: Collected Talks and Essays on Realizing God in Daily Life, Volume III* (Los Angeles: Self-Realization Fellowship, 1997).

2. Paramahansa Yogananda, *Where There Is Light: Insight and Inspiration for Meeting Life's Challenges* (Los Angeles: Self Realization Fellowship, 2015), 84.

3. Paramahansa Yogananda, *Man's Eternal Quest: Collected Talks and Essays on Realizing God in Daily Life, Volume I* (Los Angeles: Self-Realization Fellowship, 1975).

4. Pascual-Leone, et al., "Modulation of Muscle Responses Evoked by Transcranial Magnetic Stimulation During the Acquisition of New Fine Motor Skills," *Journal of Neurophysiology* 74, no. 3 (1995): 1037–1045.

5. Paramahansa Yogananda, *Scientific Healing Affirmations* (Los Angeles: Self-Realization Fellowship, 1929).

6. Margie Warrell, "How to Best Self-Doubt and Stop Selling Yourself Short," *Forbes*, December 9, 2017, https://www.forbes.com/sites/margiewarrell/2017/12/09/doubt-your-doubts/?sh=2480141b151a.

Chapter 18

1. Paramahansa Yogananda, *Autobiography of a Yogi* (Los Angeles: Self-Realization Fellowship, 1946).
2. Paramahansa Yogananda, *Cosmic Chants* (Los Angeles: Self-Realization Fellowship, 1974).
3. Ibid.
4. Ibid.
5. Paramahansa Yogananda, *Journey to Self-Realization: Collected Talks and Essays on Realizing God in Daily Life, Volume III* (Los Angeles: Self-Realization Fellowship, 1997), 280.

Chapter 19

1. Paramahansa Yogananda, *Man's Eternal Quest: Collected Talks and Essays on Realizing God in Daily Life,* Volume I (Los Angeles: Self-Realization Fellowship, 1975).
2. Paramahansa Yogananda, *Journey to Self-Realization: Collected Talks and Essays on Realizing God in Daily Life, Volume III* (Los Angeles: Self-Realization Fellowship, 1997).
3. Paramahansa Yogananda, *God Talks with Arjuna: The Bhagavad Gita.* (Los Angeles: Self-Realization Fellowship, 1995).
4. Paramahansa Yogananda, *Highest Achievements Through Self-Realization* (Los Angeles: Self-Realization Fellowship, 2019).
5. Paramahansa Yogananda, *Man's Eternal Quest: Collected Talks and Essays on Realizing God in Daily Life, Volume I* (Los Angeles: Self-Realization Fellowship, 1975).
6. Paramahansa Yogananda, *The Law of Success* (Los Angeles: Self-Realization Fellowship, 1989).
7. https://www.goodreads.com/author/quotes/22033.Brian_Tracy
8. Paramahansa Yogananda, *Journey to Self-Realization: Collected Talks and Essays on Realizing God in Daily Life, Volume III* (Los Angeles: Self-Realization Fellowship, 1997).
9. "What You Need to Know About Willpower: The Psychological Science of Self-Control," American Psychological Association, 2012, https://www.apa.org/topics/willpower.
10. Paramahansa Yogananda, *The Divine Romance: Collected Talks and Essays on Realizing God in Daily Life, Volume II* (Los Angeles: Self-Realization Fellowship, 1986).
11. Srinivasan Pillay, "Is There Scientific Evidence for the 'Law of Attraction'?" HuffPost, November 17, 2011,

https://www.huffpost.com/entry/is-there-scientific-evide_b_175189#:~:text=Recent%20brain%20imaging%20studies%20are,discovery%20of%20%22mirror%20neurons%22.&text=Our%20actions%20cause%20similar%20action%2Drepresentations%20in%20the%20brains%20of%20others.

12. Ibid.

13. Ibid.

14. Ibid.

15. Ibid.

16. Paramahansa Yogananda, *The Second Coming of Christ: The Resurrection of the Christ Within You, Discourse 32* (Los Angeles: Self-Realization Fellowship, 2004).

17. Paramahansa Yogananda, *The Divine Romance: Collected Talks and Essays on Realizing God in Daily Life, Volume II* (Los Angeles: Self-Realization Fellowship, 1986).

18. Askvik, et al., "The Importance of Cursive Handwriting over Typewriting for Learning in the Classroom: A High-Density EEG Study of 12-Year-Old Children and Young Adults," *Frontiers in Psychology* 28 (July 2020). https://doi.org/10.3389/fpsyg.2020.01810.

19. Paramahansa Yogananda, *Man's Eternal Quest: Collected Talks and Essays on Realizing God in Daily Life, Volume I* (Los Angeles: Self-Realization Fellowship, 1982), 409.

20. Paramahansa Yogananda, *Journey to Self-Realization: Collected Talks and Essays on Realizing God in Daily Life, Volume III* (Los Angeles: Self-Realization Fellowship, 1997), 380.

21. Ibid., 280.

Chapter 20

1. Paramahansa Yogananda, *God Talks with Arjuna: The Bhagavad Gita.* (Los Angeles: Self-Realization Fellowship, 1995).

2. Ibid., 427.

3. Ibid., 434.

4. Ibid., 243.

5. Paramahansa Yogananda, *Where There Is Light: Insight and Inspiration for Meeting Life's Challenges* (Los Angeles: Self-Realization Fellowship, 2015), 23.

Chapter 21

1. Paramahansa Yogananda, *Man's Eternal Quest: Collected Talks and Essays on Realizing God in Daily Life,* Volume I (Los Angeles: Self-Realization Fellowship, 1982).

ACKNOWLEDGMENTS

My deepest gratitude is first and foremost for Guruji Paramahansa Yogananda. Thank you for all the amazing teachings you have brought into the world to help guide our lives back to truth. It has been one of the greatest honors of my life to highlight them here in this book. There are no words to express my profound thankfulness and appreciation for you.

I am incredibly grateful to Hay House for believing in me and supporting me in co-creating the vision of this book into reality. In particular, I want to thank Reid Tracy, Patty Gift, and Allison Janice for getting behind me from the start! And sincere thanks to my wonderful, dedicated editor, Melody Guy, for her expert advice on the manuscript and her never-ending support for the project. Thank you to Tricia Breidenthal and the rest of the design team for helping to put form to this vision!

Enormous thanks to my dear friend, the writer Gary Jansen, for being an invaluable and tireless resource for me to bounce ideas off of and have countless hours of spiritual discourse and discussion. Gary, you are one of my dearest soul friends, and I can't thank you enough for always being there as a rock of support. You are an amazing human!

Huge thank you to the Self-Realization Fellowship for providing so much support for this book. I am incredibly grateful to Brother Satyananda for being there for me in such big ways over the years, and Lauren Landress, for tirelessly reviewing the manuscript and ensuring the accuracy of Yogananda's teachings and quotes.

I am so grateful for having the best team to run Solluna, which really feels like family. John Pisani has been my business partner since day 1, and he is also my best friend and godfather to my children. John, I cannot adequately express the depth of my gratitude for you. Thank you, thank you for always being there for me. Katelyn Hughes has also been with me for years, and she is our warrior Earth Mama for good that I love and appreciate to the moon and back! Thank you to Nicol Komitz and all our other amazing Solluna superstars that show up every day in love and dedication for the community! Deep gratitude for Casey Endo, Bianca Busketta, and Brittany Marshak, our amazing PR team that I adore.

I am so thankful for Laura Pringle, my soul sister, and intuitive healer, who has been there with me in the deepest ways that a human really can be for another. I am so incredibly grateful for you!

I am infinitely grateful for our Solluna community, all the readers and members that I am so honored to be with on this journey (including through cyberspace!). Wow! You are all amazing and you inspire me every day. I am so grateful for you and for our beautiful connection.

There are so many friends and authors who I am thankful for and who have influenced me over the years, especially Deepak Chopra and Dr. David R. Hawkins.

I am grateful to you Mick, for being on the journey of growth with me. And so thankful for my amazing parents, Bruce and Sally, for holding space for this soul along this incredible journey. And I am very grateful for Auntie Lourdes, who lived with us from birth until I was a teenager and is a human who truly embodies pure love. Thank you for loving me so much.

I am so grateful for my sons, Emerson and Moses, who are my tiny teachers of unconditional love and presence. My heart has burst open since I have been honored to become your mother.

And finally, last but not least, I want to thank my beloved husband, Jon, my King, my Rama. You are my soul mate, and you have helped me grow, clarify, and live my soul's purpose. You are a force of love and Bliss, and I am beyond grateful that we found each other. I love you.

ABOUT THE AUTHOR

KIMBERLY SNYDER is a spiritual guide, meditation teacher, nutritionist, and holistic wellness expert. She is the three-time *New York Times* best-selling author of five previous books, including *Radical Beauty*, which she co-authored with Deepak Chopra. Kimberly hosts the top-rated *Feel Good* podcast. She is the founder of Solluna®, a holistic lifestyle brand that offers wellness products, digital courses, Practical Enlightenment Meditation™, and the Solluna Circle. She has been featured in dozens of media outlets, including *Good Morning America*, *The Today Show*, and *The Wall Street Journal*. She lives in Los Angeles and Hawaii with her husband and her sons. To learn more about Kimberly and Solluna, visit: @_kimberlysnyder and www.mysolluna.com.

Hay House Titles of Related Interest

YOU CAN HEAL YOUR LIFE, the movie,
starring Louise Hay & Friends
(available as an online streaming video)
www.hayhouse.com/louise-movie

THE SHIFT, the movie,
starring Dr. Wayne W. Dyer
(available as an online streaming video)
www.hayhouse.com/the-shift-movie

***

*ALONG THE PATH TO ENLIGHTENMENT: 365 Daily
Reflections from David R. Hawkins,* edited by Scott Jeffrey

*DIVINE MASTERS, ANCIENT WISDOM: Activations
to Connect with Universal Spiritual Guides,* by Kyle Gray

*THE LIFE OF YOGANANDA: The Story of the Yogi Who
Became the First Modern Guru,* by Philip Goldberg

*POWER VS. FORCE: The Hidden Determinants
of Human Behavior,* by Dr. David R. Hawkins

YOGA, POWER & SPIRIT: Patanjali the Shaman,
by Alberto Villoldo, Ph.D.

All of the above are available at your local bookstore,
or may be ordered by contacting Hay House (see next page).

***

We hope you enjoyed this Hay House book. If you'd like to receive our online catalog featuring additional information on Hay House books and products, or if you'd like to find out more about the Hay Foundation, please contact:

Hay House, Inc., P.O. Box 5100, Carlsbad, CA 92018-5100
(760) 431-7695 or (800) 654-5126
(760) 431-6948 (fax) or (800) 650-5115 (fax)
www.hayhouse.com® • www.hayfoundation.org

———

Published in Australia by: Hay House Australia Pty. Ltd.,
18/36 Ralph St., Alexandria NSW 2015
Phone: 612-9669-4299 • *Fax:* 612-9669-4144
www.hayhouse.com.au

Published in the United Kingdom by: Hay House UK, Ltd.,
The Sixth Floor, Watson House, 54 Baker Street, London W1U 7BU
Phone: +44 (0)20 3927 7290 • *Fax:* +44 (0)20 3927 7291
www.hayhouse.co.uk

Published in India by: Hay House Publishers India,
Muskaan Complex, Plot No. 3, B-2, Vasant Kunj, New Delhi 110 070
Phone: 91-11-4176-1620 • *Fax:* 91-11-4176-1630
www.hayhouse.co.in

———

Access New Knowledge.
Anytime. Anywhere.

Learn and evolve at your own pace
with the world's leading experts.

www.hayhouseU.com

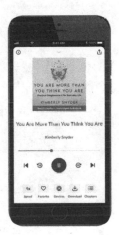

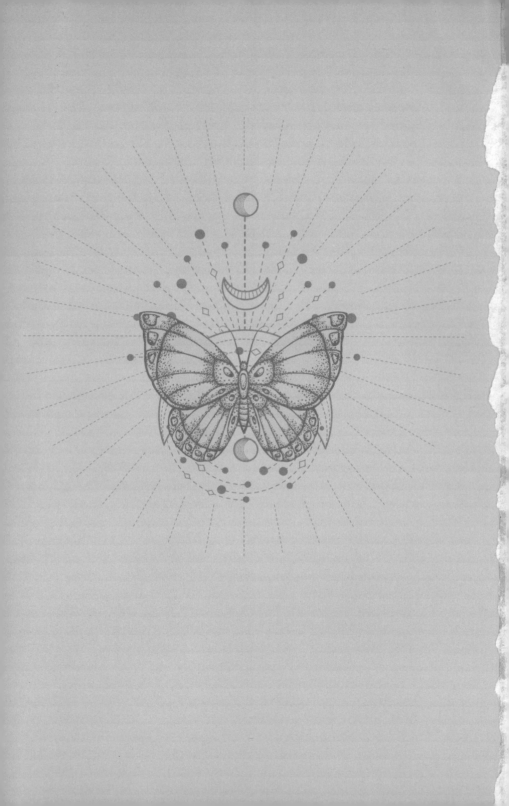